Blueprints

**CLINICAL CASES
NEUROLOGY,
2nd EDITION**

Check Out all the Titles in This Great Series!

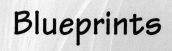

Blueprints

CLINICAL CASES

SECOND EDITION

NEUROLOGY

Kevin N. Sheth, MD
Chief Resident, Department of Neurology
Massachusetts General Hospital
Brigham and Women's Hospital
Harvard Medical School
Boston, Massachusetts

Odette A. Harris, MD, MPH
Assistant Professor, Department of Neurosurgery
Emory University
Chief of Service, Neurosurgery
Grady Memorial Hospital

Tracey A. Cho, MD, MA
Chief Resident, Department of Neurology
Massachusetts General Hospital
Brigham and Women's Hospital
Harvard Medical School
Boston, Massachusetts

Aaron B. Caughey, MD, MPP, MPH, PHD (Series Editor)
Assistant Professor, Division of Perinatal Medicine and Genetics
Department of Obstetrics & Gynecology
University of California, San Francisco
San Francisco, California

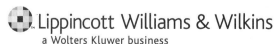

Lippincott Williams & Wilkins
a Wolters Kluwer business
Philadelphia · Baltimore · New York · London
Buenos Aires · Hong Kong · Sydney · Tokyo

Acquisitions Editor: Nancy Anastasi Duffy
Managing Editor: Stacey L. Sebring
Marketing Manager: Jennifer Kuklinski
Associate Production Manager: Kevin P. Johnson
Creative Director: Doug Smock
Compositor: International Typesetting and Composition
Printer: R.R. Donnelley & Son's

Printed in the United States of America

First Edition, 2002
Second Edition, 2007

Library of Congress Cataloging-in-Publication Data

Sheth, Kevin.
   Blueprints clinical cases in neurology / Kevin Sheth, Odette A. Harris,
Tracey A. Cho. — 2nd ed.
       p. ; cm. — (Blueprints. Clinical cases)
   Rev. ed. of: Blueprints clinical cases in neurology / Sucheta M. Joshi.
2002.
   Includes bibliographical references and index.
   ISBN-13: 978-1-4051-0494-4
   ISBN-10: 1-4051-0494-5
  1. Neurology—Case studies. I. Harris, Odette A. II. Cho, Tracey A.
III. Joshi, Sucheta M. Blueprints clinical cases in neurology. IV. Title.
V. Title: Clinical cases in neurology. VI. Series.
   [DNLM: 1. Nervous System Diseases—diagnosis—Case Reports. 2. Nervous
System Diseases—diagnosis—Problems and Exercises. 3. Diagnosis,
Differential—Case Reports. 4. Diagnosis, Differential—Problems and
Exercises. WL 18.2 S554b 2007]
RC359.J67 2007
616.80076—dc22
                                                                2006015073

The publishers have made every effort to trace the copyright holders for borrowed material. If they have inadvertently overlooked any, they will be pleased to make the necessary arrangements at the first opportunity.

07 08 09 10
2 3 4 5 6 7 8 9 10

Dedication

To my brother, Kinjal, my parents, Sucheta and Navin, for their love and to Joshua Levine, my friend and teacher for inspiring me in the first place.

Kevin

To my husband, Edward, and to my family, for their continued love and support.

Odette

We would all like to thank the staff at Blackwell Publishing and now Lippincott William & Wilkins for their work to improve and polish this book. I would also like to thank my family, friends, and colleagues for their support for my many endeavors. This book is dedicated to the memory of my grandfather, Theodore Schraft.

Aaron

To my wife, Josalyn, for all of your love and support.

Tracey

Preface

The *Blueprints Clinical Cases* series has been written to complement clinical rotations in neurology, and to serve as preparation material for the boards or in-service examinations. In compiling these cases, we have tried to cover common conditions in neurology as are encountered in the clinic, ward, and emergency room.

The format of the book has been designed to parallel actual clinical experience, and is therefore different from the more usual case-presentation and multiple-choice-questions format. One of the aspects of clinical medicine unique to neurology is lesion localization. Several of the cases have been designed with lesion localization as the central part of the thinking process.

This book does not cover every neurologic condition, but addresses common diseases. We have included common neurosurgical topics and topics from pediatric neurology as well. There are a few zebras, but by and large common topics have been addressed. The principal goal of these cases is to stimulate thinking about a disease process, localizing anatomic lesions and physiologic processes, rather than enumerating tests and treatments for a given condition. The book is not meant to be a textbook of neurology, and the reader should make use of *Blueprints Clinical Cases in Neurology* as well as standard textbooks for reference.

CASE FORMAT

Chief Complaint/ID: This describes the complaint that brings the patient to medical attention. When you read the chief complaint or even just the case title, you should begin to think of a differential and how you would differentiate between diagnoses.

Medical History: A brief history with onset and progression of symptoms is described. This also includes medication history, allergies, and social and family histories. Review of this section should suggest broad categories of differential diagnoses and begin to help you rule out aspects of your differential from the chief complaint.

Physical Examination: The physical examination represents pertinent positives and negatives. Because the neurologic examination is imperative in focusing the differential, it is presented at great length in many of the cases. While an imaging study will often help to pinpoint a lesion, the neurologic examination, historically, has been quite accurate as well.

Thought Questions: These open-ended questions are meant to stimulate ideas regarding lesion localization and pathophysiology. To get the most out of these questions, spend some time reflecting on possible answers. For most cases, this is the cornerstone of the case, as it deals with lesion localization. Lesion localization helps formulate a hypothesis and design a patient's work-up. Answers to the thought questions follow.

Case Continuation: After discussion of the thought questions, the case is continued with examination findings where necessary, relevant work-up, and results. For some cases, there may be more thought questions; some cases conclude at this point.

Questions: Each case is followed by multiple-choice questions. The questions address the condition itself, aspects of relevant basic anatomy or physiology, and treatment principles. In some cases even clinical aspects of the cases not alluded to in the body of the case are touched upon in the questions. The answers are not all-inclusive, so further reading is recommended.

Approach the cases as you would approach a patient. Some of the cases have been written in a rather informal format, to mimic how patients describe the history during an interview. Most cases are inspired by real patients and experiences; some have been simplified keeping the audience in mind.

Case-based learning is an integral part of medicine, and perhaps the most enjoyable way to learn it. We hope that students, sub-interns, and even junior physicians enjoy thinking about these cases as much as we enjoyed putting them together.

We have made exciting additions and changes to the second edition that we believe will enhance the experience on the wards, preparation for boards and in-service examinations, and care of a variety of neurologic patients. We have included references with each case to provide the reader with an up-to-date guide of the latest trials and therapies. Additionally, we have added a section of stand-alone questions. This question and answer section serves to simulate questions that may appear on national neurology examinations for medical students and residents.

We hope that, through these cases, you will come to share the excitement of neurology with us.

Kevin N. Sheth
Odette A. Harris
Tracey A. Cho
Aaron B. Caughey

Acknowledgments

We would like to acknowledge the work of Drs. Sucheta Joshi and Annette Langer-Gould in the first edition of this book. Additionally, our thanks to Drs. Jin S. Hahn, Donald M. Olson, and Ross Goldstein, Stanford University Medical Center, for helping find images to illustrate cases. Thanks to Beth Hoyt, Stanford University Medical Center, for compiling images from scans into illustrations.

Contents

Abbreviations/Acronyms

ALS	amyotrophic lateral sclerosis
Baso	basophils
BBB	blood-brain barrier
BP	blood pressure
BUN	blood urea nitrogen
C	cervical
CABG	coronary artery bypass graft
CAD	coronary artery disease
CBC	complete blood count
CC	chief complaint
CIDP	chronic inflammatory demyelinating polyneuropathy
CK	creatine kinase
CMV	cytomegalovirus
CN	cranial nerve
CNS	central nervous system
COPD	chronic obstructive pulmonary disease
COR	coronary exam
CPAP	continuous positive airway pressure
CSF	cerebrospinal fluid
CT	computed tomography
CTA	clear to auscultation
CVA	cerebrovascular accident
CXR	chest radiograph
DMD	Duchenne (de Boulogne) muscular dystrophy
Dz	disease
ECHO	echocardiography
ECG	electrocardiogram
ED	emergency department
EEG	electroencephalogram
EMG	electromyogram
ENT	ear, nose, and throat
EOMI	extraocular movements intact
Eos	eosinophils
ER	emergency room
ESR	erythrocyte sedimentation rate
EtOH	ethanol

FANA	fluorescent anti-nuclear antibody
FHx	family history
FTA	fluorescent treponemal antibody
Gen	general
Glc	glucose
HA	headache
HD	heart disease
HDL	high density lipoprotein
HEENT	head, eyes, ears, nose, and throat
HIV	human immunodeficiency virus
HLA	human leukocyte antigen
HR	heart rate
HRT	hormone replacement therapy
HTN	hypertension
H & P	history and physical
ICU	intensive care unit
ID	identification
INR	international normalized ratio
IV	intravenous
IVDA	intravenous drug abuse
L	lumbar
LDL	low density lipoprotein
LEMS	Lambert-Eaton myasthenic syndrome
LFTs	liver function tests
LMN	lower motor neuron
LP	lumbar puncture
Lymphs	lymphocytes
MAO	monoamine oxidase
MCA	middle cerebral artery
MDI	metered-dose inhaler
MEDS	medications
MG	myasthenia gravis
MID	multi-infarct dementia
MMSE	Mini Mental Status Examination
Monos	monocytes
MRI	magnetic resonance imaging
NCV	nerve conduction velocity
Neuro	neurologic
Neuro Hx	neurologic history
Neuts	neutrophils
NKDA	no known drug allergies
NSAID	nonsteroidal anti-inflammatory drug
NT	nontender
N & V	nausea and vomiting

OB	obstetrician
OFC	occipital-frontal circumference
OTC	over-the-counter
PCR	polymerase chain reaction
PE	physical examination
PERRLA	pupils equal, round, and reactive to light and accommodation
PET	positron emission tomography
PMHx	past medical history
PML	progressive multifocal leukoencephalopathy
PMN	polymorphonuclear cells
PPD	pack per day
PSHx	past surgical history
PT	prothrombin time
PTC	pseudotumor cerebri
PTT	partial thromboplastin time
RBC	red blood cell
RRR	regular rate and rhythm
SAH	subarachnoid hemorrhage
SE	status epilepticus
SHx	social history
TFT	thyroid function tests
TG	triglycerides
Th	thoracic
TIA	transient ischemic attack
TSH	thyroid stimulating hormone
UMN	upper motor neuron
URI	upper respiratory tract infection
VP	ventriculoperitoneal
VS	vital signs
WBC	white blood cell
WBRT	whole brain radiation therapy
WNL	within normal limits

I

Patients Who Present with a Seizure

Seizure

ID/CC: 37-year-old woman with new-onset seizure.

HPI: NS experienced a seizure while at work. The event was witnessed by a colleague who is a retired nurse. NS recovered from the event without any neurologic sequelae and was brought directly to the ER. She and her colleague describe the event as repeated jerking of her left arm. The movements were rapid at first, but over the course of approximately 3 minutes, they slowed and eventually ceased. Ms. S was sweating during the event. There was no noted aura and no incontinence. She remained conscious throughout the entire event.

PMHx: Asthma, no history of seizures, trauma, or CNS infection

PSHx: None

Meds: MDI, as needed

All: NKDA

FHx: No history of intracranial tumors, no seizure history

SHx: Married mother of two children. Works as an engineer.

Habits: No tobacco, occasional alcohol, no IVDA or recreational drugs

VS: Temp 99.1°F BP 130/80 HR 78 RR 12

PE/Neuro: The examination is entirely WNL

Labs/drug screen: WNL

THOUGHT QUESTIONS

- Does the patient have epilepsy?
- What is the differential diagnosis?

NS experienced a new-onset seizure. In the evaluation of new seizures, it is important to determine whether a seizure has actually occurred. The occurrence of loss of consciousness or jerking movements is not in itself diagnostic. The history given, corroborated by a retired nurse, seems consistent with a simple partial seizure. A seizure may be defined as a transient disturbance of cerebral function caused by an abnormal neuronal discharge. Seizures may manifest in numerous ways and may result from a variety of causes. Epilepsy, simply defined, is characterized by recurrent seizures. In this case such a diagnosis is inappropriate.

The differential diagnosis of the patient presented must stem from her presenting issue of new-onset seizures. Etiologies include, but are not limited to: metabolic abnormalities—hyponatremia, hypocalcemia, hypoglycemia, hypomagnesemia and uremia; systemic diseases—hypertensive encephalopathy, hepatic encephalopathy, and hyperthermia; CNS dysfunction—trauma, stroke, mass lesion; drugs—alcohol withdrawal and intoxicants; and idiopathic causes. The patient's laboratory studies and history allow us to remove from the differential metabolic abnormalities, drugs and most systemic diseases.

CASE CONTINUED

Subsequent evaluation, including noncontrast and contrast CT and MRI of the head, revealed a 2-cm right-sided convexity (near the coronal suture) mass. The lesion is well demarcated, intensely enhancing with a prominent dural tail. No other intracranial abnormalities were identified.

THOUGHT QUESTIONS

- What is your differential diagnosis?
- Is this a case of sporadic meningioma or is there evidence to support it being familial?
- What aspects of the history are inconsistent with neurofibromatosis?
- Is the history of seizure inconsistent with the diagnosis of meningioma?

The differential diagnosis at this time is narrowed to CNS-mass lesion. The imaging characteristics, although not pathognomonic, are highly suggestive of a meningioma. When coupled with the history and PE, other possibilities are far less likely. Meningiomas account for approximately 15% of primary intracranial tumors. They are more commonly found in women with a female-to-male ratio ranging from 2:1 to 4:1.

Most meningiomas are incidentally identified as less than 10% present because of symptoms. If symptomatic, seizures and hemiparesis are frequently associated with convexity-based lesions. This case is consistent with a sporadic case of meningioma. Most meningiomas fall into this category of isolated lesions. The familial type is also known as neurofibromatosis type 2 (NF-2). Such a diagnosis would depend on the presence of bilateral acoustic neuromas, or a first-degree relative with a diagnosis of NF-2 and the presence of a single acoustic neuroma, or any two of the following: schwannoma, meningioma, acoustic neuroma, neurofibroma, glioma, or juvenile postsubcapsular lens opacity. The family history, PE and radiographic findings are all inconsistent with this diagnosis.

 CASE CONTINUED

The lesion is surgically resected. There are no intra-operative complications. The pathologist has confirmed a typical meningioma, with psammoma bodies and whorls, that is both epithelial membrane antigen (EMA) and vimentin positive.

QUESTIONS

1-1. Which of the following pathology findings are concerning for malignancy?
- A. EMA positive
- B. Vimentin positive
- C. Presence of psammoma bodies
- D. None of the above

1-2. Meningiomas arise from which of the following?
A. Osteocytes
B. The vascular supply of the dura
C. Arachnoid cap cells
D. None of the above

1-3. Which of the following is specific for the malignant group of meningiomas?
A. The presence of a dural tail
B. Hypercellularity
C. Metastases
D. Invasion of the brain

1-4. The two most common cranial locations of meningiomas are:
A. Convexity and orbital groove
B. Convexity and parasagittal
C. Foramen magnum and olfactory groove
D. Sphenoid wing and olfactory groove

ANSWERS

1-1. D. The findings of psammoma bodies and whorls that are both EMA and vimentin positive are consistent with "typical," nonmalignant meningioma. This is the most common type, accounting for 92% of meningiomas. EMA helps to distinguish meningioma from other types of tumor, such as schwannoma. It does not distinguish between typical and more aggressive forms of meningioma. Although these features are present in the malignant type of meningioma, their presence alone is in no way concerning for malignancy and does not affect prognosis. (See also answer to question 3.)

1-2. C. Meningiomas arise from arachnoid cap cells, not the dura, or osteocytes.

1-3. D. The presence of a dural tail is suggestive of meningioma, but is not diagnostic. It has no prognostic value. Hypercellularity, increased mitoses, necrosis, and metastases are not specific to the malignant group and may also be found in the "atypical" group. Brain invasion is specific for the malignant group of meningioma.

1-4. B. Although meningioma may occur in any of the listed locations, parasagittal and convexity (near the coronal suture) meningiomas are the two most common intracranial locations.

SUGGESTED ADDITIONAL READING

Browne TR, Holmes GL. Primary care: epilepsy. N Engl J Med 2001;344:1145–1151.

Chang BS, Lowenstein DH. Mechanisms of disease: epilepsy. N Engl J Med 2003;349:1257–1266.

New Onset Seizure in Adulthood

 ID/CC: 45-year-old woman presents with new onset seizures and altered consciousness.

HPI: TC was talking to a coworker when she suddenly stared, turned her head to the right, began smacking her lips, and then had a generalized tonic-clonic seizure. The seizure lasted 2 to 3 minutes. Ms. C does not recall anything immediately prior to or during the event and was still confused 20 minutes later. Her husband and a coworker state that she has not been physically ill recently but over the last 2 months has been "having a mid-life crisis."

PMHx: None

PSHx: None

Meds: None

All: NKDA

SHx: Graphic designer, married with one daughter. Recently decided she wanted a divorce despite lack of marital conflict. Drinks one glass of wine a day.

FHX: HTN

Neuro Hx: None

THOUGHT QUESTIONS

- What is your differential diagnosis? (at least three possibilities)
- What signs will you look for on examination and what laboratory tests will you order to aid in diagnosis?

The differential diagnosis is an isolated partial seizure, primary (idiopathic) epilepsy, or a partial seizure secondary to intoxication/withdrawal, underlying metabolic disorder, infection, or structural lesion.

The work-up for secondary causes of seizures in this case includes a screen for toxins, comprehensive metabolic panel including Ca^{++} and Mg^{++}, CBC for evidence of systemic infection or anemia, LP for evidence of a CNS infection, and a CT or MRI scan to rule out an underlying structural lesion. An EEG may be useful, particularly if the prior work-up is unrevealing, but is not necessary in the acute setting in this patient.

CASE CONTINUED

VS: Temp 98.6°F BP 110/70 HR 76 RR 16

PE: Gen: No rashes.

MSE: Initially patient responds only to simple commands and is unable to converse but over the course of your examination she improves dramatically and complains of a bifrontal HA. She tells you that she had a minor sore throat over the last week and maybe a low-grade temperature although she never measured it. She denies having any prior headaches or seizures. When asked about any changes in mood she denies this and says that she has not been depressed but feels that she needs to be free to pursue her dream of becoming a movie star. She plans on divorcing her husband and moving to Los Angeles "to be discovered." She has no training or experience as an actress, does not plan on going to acting school, and has never performed in a play since grade school. She denies any hallucinations.

Neuro: CN II–XII: Intact

Fundi: No papilledema. Visual fields are full.

Motor: Normal bulk, tone, and strength to direct muscle testing

Reflexes: 2+ throughout. Babinski signs present bilaterally.

Sensory: Intact to light touch, vibration, pinprick, and temperature sensation throughout

Coordination: No tremor, dysmetria, or dysdiadochokinesis.

Gait: No ataxia, intact tandem gait.

Labs: CBC, comprehensive metabolic panel, and toxic screen are all WNL.

**Imaging
Studies:**   CT scan shows a poorly circumscribed, hypointense left temporal lobe lesion with small foci of hemorrhage and possible early uncal herniation, with minimal surrounding edema.

 QUESTIONS

   2-1. What is the most likely diagnosis?
      A. Herpes simplex viral encephalitis
      B. Metastatic tumor
      C. Primary brain tumor
      D. Stroke

   2-2. How should you proceed?
      A. Obtain an MRI
      B. Perform an LP
      C. Load with IV phenytoin
      D. Start IV acyclovir

   2-3. Over the next week the patient remains stable. Her MRI shows a large, poorly circumscribed cortical, left temporal lobe lesion with areas of hemorrhage and necrosis. The uncal herniation is mild with no evidence of brainstem compression. The lesion is biopsied. What is the most likely result of her biopsy?
      A. Healed inflammatory lesions and viral inclusion bodies
      B. Oligodendroglioma
      C. Malignant glioma
      D. Primary CNS lymphoma

   2-4. Which of the following treatments is avoided to most likely prolong her survival or improve her quality of life?
      A. Extensive surgical resection
      B. Antiepileptics
      C. Radiotherapy
      D. Systemic chemotherapy
      E. Corticosteroids

ANSWERS

2-1. C. The most likely diagnosis is a primary brain tumor. The insidious onset of personality changes, the lack of fixed deficits on examination, a poorly circumscribed unilateral temporal lobe lesion, and return to her baseline mentation all suggest that this is a subacute rather than acute process. Herpes simplex virus (HSV) encephalitis usually presents with bilateral orbitofrontal or bitemporal lesions and is rarely unilateral. Additionally, HSV encephalitis is accompanied by systemic signs of infection such as fever and elevated WBC. Metastatic tumors are typically well circumscribed with significant surrounding edema. The subacute onset of symptoms and lack of fixed deficit on exam make a cerebral infarct extremely unlikely. If this were a stroke the CT abnormalities should also follow a vascular rather than a cortical distribution.

2-2. A. This patient has evidence of uncal herniation on CT scan and thus an LP may precipitate a potentially fatal herniation syndrome. An oral load with phenytoin or carbamazepine would suffice because the patient is not in status epilepticus. IV phenytoin can occasionally cause necrosis at the infusion site and thus poses an unnecessary risk in this patient. MRI would be helpful in identifying any occult disease of the opposite hemisphere not seen on CT scan and any possible early brainstem compression signs associated with the uncal herniation.

2-3. C. Malignant glioma is the most common primary brain tumor in adults. The frontal and temporal lobes are the most frequent sites of involvement. Oligodendrogliomas are rare and usually have areas of partial calcification, which would have been evident on the CT scan. Primary CNS lymphoma usually occurs in immunocompromised individuals although the incidence in non-immunocompromised people has been increasing. When presenting as an intraparenchymal tumor, the lesions usually appear in the periventricular areas and basal ganglia, are well circumscribed, enhance diffusely, and have significant peritumoral edema.

2-4. D. The combination of extensive surgical resection and radiotherapy doubles the median survival (from 17 to 38 weeks) and provides symptomatic relief. A surgical cure is very rare, because gliomas are highly invasive and most have already micrometastasized at the time of diagnosis. Control of seizures and increased intracranial pressure from peritumoral edema using antiepileptics and corticosteroids, respectively, will improve quality of life. Systemic chemotherapy is likely to diminish her quality of life and does not lead to any significant improvement in survival.

 ADDITIONAL SUGGESTED READING

Berg AT, Shinnar S. The risk of seizure recurrence following a first unprovoked seizure: a quantitative review. Neurology 1991;41:965.
Kosten TR, O'Connor PG. Current concepts: management of drug and alcohol withdrawal. N Engl J Med 2003;348:1786–1795.

Prolonged Seizures

 ID/CC: 52-year-old man with seizures

HPI: BS is a 52-year-old male brought into the ED by paramedics. Earlier the patient's wife called 911 reporting that the patient had a seizure and was unresponsive after it. When paramedics arrived at the scene, the patient was having another generalized tonic-clonic seizure, and the wife confirmed that it had begun just after she got off the phone and that the seizure had not stopped.

En route to the ED, the paramedics administered a single dose of IV diazepam, which produced little effect. The patient was brought into the ED, still seizing

PMHx: History of epilepsy, secondary to head trauma 5 years ago

PSHx: Tonsillectomy at age 7

Med: Carbamazepine (long-acting formulation) 400 mg BID, multivitamin daily

All: Phenobarbital

SHx: Former factory manager, now unemployed because of his epilepsy. Married, wife works as a legal secretary

VS: Temp 99.3°F BP 130/85 HR 108 RR 18

PE: Gen: Sinus tachycardia, scar on right parietal region of scalp from previous head trauma

Mental status: Lethargic, minimally responsive to pain

Cranial nerves: Constricted but reactive pupils, otherwise unremarkable

Motor: No obvious focal deficits

Reflexes: Brisk muscle stretch reflexes on the left, extensor plantar response on the left. He also has intermittent subtle twitching of his left eyelid, face, and arm.

THOUGHT QUESTIONS

- What is status epilepticus?
- Is an EEG mandatory to make the diagnosis?

Status epilepticus (SE) is a neurologic emergency. It is the occurrence of seizures that persist for a sufficient length of time without recovery between seizures. This may be a single prolonged seizure or repeated seizures without recovery of consciousness between two seizures. SE can be generalized SE or partial SE, depending upon the type of seizures. In the early stages seizures may be clinically obvious in SE, but as SE is prolonged, the manifestations of seizures may be subtle (such as subtle clonic jerking or eye deviation). SE should be differentiated from acute repetitive or serial seizures where consciousness is preserved between seizures.

Electroencephalography is not required to make the diagnosis of SE. Treatment of SE should not wait for an EEG, as valuable time will be lost in doing so, and treatment of SE must begin promptly.

CASE CONTINUED

Labs: CBC: WBC 12,000/mm³, with 54% neutrophils, rest of CBC WNL. Chemistries including glucose, LFTs, BUN, Cr WNL. Carbamazepine level: 2.5 µg/mL (therapeutic range 8 to 12 µg/mL)

THOUGHT QUESTION

- How will you proceed with treatment of SE?

Treatment of SE involves initial "ABCs" common to all emergencies, a focused history and PE and prompt measures to stop seizures. The initial treatment should include IV dextrose and thiamine. This is followed by rapid institution of anticonvulsant therapy.

Initial anticonvulsant therapy involves use of a benzodiazepine such as diazepam or lorazepam. After administration of a benzodiazepine, a longer-acting agent is administered. Phenytoin sodium intravenously is the drug of choice. Dose: bolus infusion of 18 mg/kg, given at an infusion rate not exceeding 50 mg/minute. Fosphenytoin, a more recently available prodrug of phenytoin, can be given at a faster infusion rate (150 mg/minute), and does not cause as much irritation to peripheral veins. Both can cause infusion-rate dependent hypotension and cardiac dysrhythmias, for which the infusion is slowed down (Table 3-1).

TABLE 3-1 Outline for Treatment of Status Epilepticus

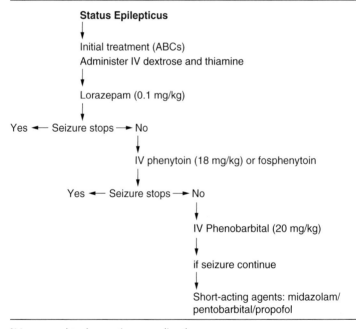

*May proceed to short-acting agent directly.

    CASE CONTINUED

The patient received a bolus of 50 mL of 50% dextrose, 100 mg of thiamine, followed by two doses of 2 mg each of lorazepam. He was then given 18 mg/kg IV fosphenytoin, and put on a maintenance dose.

Over the next 24 hours the patient had no further seizures. He became progressively more responsive, and his carbamazepine was restarted. It was later learned that he had been taking 200 mg once a day for a week prior to this episode, because of low supplies.

QUESTIONS

3-1. Etiology of SE includes
A. Stroke
B. Head trauma
C. Hepatic coma
D. All of the above
E. None of the above

3-2. Mortality in SE is approximately
A. 5%
B. 10%
C. 20%
D. 50%

3-3. Drugs used to treat SE include all of the following except:
A. Phenobarbital
B. Lorazepam
C. Phenytoin
D. Carbamazepine
E. Diazepam

3-4. Short-acting agents used in treatment of refractory SE include all except which of the following?
A. Fentanyl
B. Pentobarbital
C. Propofol
D. Midazolam

ANSWERS

3-1. D. The etiology of SE is varied and includes acute processes such as stroke, electrolyte abnormalities (including renal/hepatic failure), head trauma, drug toxicity, and CNS infections. Chronic processes include breakthrough seizures in a patient with epilepsy because of noncompliance with medications, and other acute CNS insults.

3-2. C. Mortality in SE is approximately 20%, related to the etiology of SR and consequences from SE (hypoxia, acidosis). Prompt recognition and treatment is important in reducing mortality.

3-3. D. Treatment of SE requires use of a parenteral medication. Carbamazepine is available only in oral form. It is not indicated for use in SE.

3-4. A. SE unresponsive to conventional treatment with a benzodiazepine phenytoin (phenobarbital) is considered refractory SE, and warrants treatment with a short-acting sedative/anesthetic agent. These are given as a continuous infusion, titrated to cessation of seizures or "burst-suppression" pattern on EEG within the limits of the patient's tolerance. The most common side effect from these agents is hypotension, which usually requires vasopressor support. Midazolam, pentobarbital, and propofol are short-acting agents used for this purpose. Fentanyl is a narcotic analgesic agent. While it has sedative properties, it has no role in the treatment of refractory SE.

 ADDITIONAL SUGGESTED READING

Lowenstein DH. Current concepts: status epilepticus. N Engl J Med 1998;338:970–976.

Treatment of convulsive status epilepticus. Recommendations of the Epilepsy Foundation of America's Working Group on Status Epilepticus. JAMA 1993;270:854.

New Onset Seizure and Fever

 ID/CC: 67-year-old woman presents with fever, seizures, and altered consciousness.

HPI: Patient's husband states that she had been ill over the last 2 days complaining of fever, headache, and fatigue. The morning of admission her husband tried to wake her, she was confused, incoherent, and then had two generalized tonic-clonic seizures back to back, each lasting 2 to 3 minutes and she has not regained normal mentation since then. The seizures occurred more than 1 hour ago.

PMHx: None

PSHx: None

Meds: HRT, calcium supplements, and acetaminophen over the last several days for her illness

All: NKDA

SHx: Married, homemaker, four adult children. She drinks two glasses of wine each evening.

FHx: Heart Dz

Neuro Hx: No prior history of seizures or headaches.

THOUGHT QUESTIONS

- How would you summarize the case thus far?
- What is your differential diagnosis? (at least three possibilities)
- What signs will you look for on examination and laboratory tests will you order to aid in diagnosis?

▪ Name the most common organisms responsible for bacterial meningitis in developed countries and the most common organisms in her age group.

▪ Discuss the typical CSF findings in acute bacterial meningitis and four circumstances under which these typical CSF findings may be absent.

In summarizing neurologic cases it is important to note the temporal course of the problem (acute, subacute, or chronic) and whether the symptoms are intermittent or continuous (and if so stable or progressive). The next step is to grossly localize the lesion in order to be able to generate a reasonable differential diagnosis. With this in mind the summary is as follows: A previously healthy woman develops new onset seizures and encephalopathy during an acute, febrile illness. This points to global cerebral involvement.

The differential diagnosis for acute onset of seizures and encephalopathy in the setting of a febrile illness includes encephalitis, meningitis, septic emboli, and seizures and encephalopathy because of metabolic derangements (uremia in the setting of kidney failure, hyperammonemia in the setting of acute liver failure) from acute inflammatory renal or hepatic failure. Delirium tremens or alcohol withdrawal seizures should also be considered, but is unlikely if the social history of two glasses of wine per night is correct.

Physical and laboratory examination should look for other signs of infection, kidney or liver failure, and focal neurologic deficits (weakness, sensory loss), as well as signs of meningismus and an assessment of level of consciousness.

The most common organisms causing acute bacterial meningitis in developed countries are *Haemophilus influenzae, Neisseria meningitidis, Streptococcus pneumoniae,* and gram-negative bacilli other than *H. influenzae* (most frequently *Escherichia coli, Klebsiella pneumoniae*). In people older than the age of 60 years, *S. pneumoniae, N. meningitidis*, and gram-negative bacilli are the most common.

The typical CSF findings in acute bacterial meningitis are markedly elevated cell count (predominantly polymorphonuclear cells), low glucose (less than 40 mg/dL), and an elevated protein (over 50 mg/dL). These findings can be absent in (1) immunocompromised patients; (2) atypical bacteria such as *Borrelia burgdorferi, Treponema pallidum, Listeria monocytogenes*, and *Leptospira interrogans*;

(3) early in the course of an overwhelming infection where the poly-morphonuclear response may be poor, such as with *S. pneumoniae*; and (4) in a patient with a partially treated meningitis.

CASE CONTINUED

VS: Temp 103.2°F BP 110/70 HR 120 RR 20

PE: No skin or nail lesions. COR: RRR, no murmurs. Lungs: CTA. Abdomen: soft, NT, no organomegaly.

Neuro: MSE: Agitated, responding to simple commands only, muttering incoherently

CNs: PERRLA, moves eyes conjugately in all directions, corneal reflexes present bilaterally, gag reflex intact

Motor: Moving all four limbs spontaneously

Reflexes: 2+ throughout. Babinski signs present bilaterally

Sensory: Withdraws all four limbs to touch

Coordination: No tremor or nystagmus

Gait: Patient restrained, not testable

Labs: Comprehensive metabolic panel WNL, WBC 16.4. 85% neuts, 10% lymphs, 5% monos, 2% eos, 0.3% baso, serum ammonia WNL. UA: WNL

QUESTIONS

  4-1. What is the most appropriate next step?
   A. Start IV ampicillin and IV ceftriaxone
   B. Obtain LP
   C. Start IV ampicillin, ceftriaxone, and acyclovir
   D. Start IV phenytoin
   E. Obtain a CT scan

4-2. Which additional laboratory tests should be ordered next to aid in diagnosis?
   A. LP with opening pressure
   B. Brain scan
   C. EEG
   D. Blood cultures
   E. None of the above

4-3. The LP shows opening pressure of 230 mm of H_2O, WBC = 100 cells/mm³, 65% lymphs, 35% PMNs, 10% mononuclear cells, RBC = 26,000 cells/mm³, protein = 85 mg/dL, glc = 60 mg/dL in tubes 1 and 3. What is the most likely diagnosis?
   A. Viral encephalitis
   B. Bacterial meningitis
   C. Embolic cerebral infarction with endocarditis
   D. Tuberculoid meningitis
   E. Traumatic tap

4-4. Assuming you have made the correct decisions up to this point, what is this patient's risk of mortality during the acute phase of her illness?
   A. 1%
   B. 5%
   C. 10%
   D. 40%

 ANSWERS

4-1. C. Although a diagnosis has not been established, death and permanent neurologic damage are the dangers if this patient is not treated immediately for potential bacterial meningitis and herpes encephalitis. No time should be wasted.

4-2. B. Once treatment has been initiated the patient should obtain an urgent CT scan to look for early signs of herniation, which would preclude safely proceeding with an LP. The examination of CSF is crucial in this patient for establishing a diagnosis and should be sent at minimum for a white count, protein, glucose, Gram stain, bacterial culture, and herpes simplex virus polymerase chain reaction (HSV PCR) analysis. An opening pressure should be obtained to aid in differential diagnosis and assess need for monitoring and treatment of increased intracranial pressure. A characteristic EEG finding in HSV encephalitis is bifrontal and/or bitemporal periodic lateralizing epileptiform discharges (PLEDs).

Bacterial meningitis can be associated with sepsis and blood cultures should be drawn as well.

4-3. A. Viral encephalitis is the most likely diagnosis. The LP shows an elevated opening pressure, lymphocytic pleocytosis, elevated protein, normal glucose, and elevated RBCs. In a traumatic tap the number of RBCs should decrease from tubes 1 and 3. If the number is equivalent in subsequent tubes, this indicates an SAH. The most common causes of viral encephalitis are HSV, arboviruses, mumps, and enteroviruses. SAH occurs almost exclusively with HSV encephalitis. Hemorrhagic bitemporal/bifrontal lesions are what one would expect on CT scan in this case of herpes simplex encephalitis. CSF findings in bacterial meningitis and embolic cerebral infarctions from endocarditis in a nonimmunocompromised individual are usually elevated WBCs with PMNs predominating, high protein, and low glucose. Tuberculoid meningitis usually presents as a subacute or chronic febrile meningitis and the characteristic CSF findings are a lymphocytic pleocytosis, high protein, and low glucose.

4-4. C. The risk of mortality during the acute phase of clinically recognized viral encephalitis is 10%. If acyclovir treatment is delayed in HSV encephalitis patients, mortality may be as high as 40%. The risk of serious residual deficits, such as memory loss, aphasia, and personality changes, are high even if appropriate treatment is instituted early.

 ADDITIONAL SUGGESTED READING

Quagliarello VJ, Scheld WM. Treatment of bacterial meningitis. N Engl J Med 1997;336:708–716.

van de Beek D, de Gans J, Spanjaard L, et al. Clinical features and prognostic factors in adults with bacterial meningitis. N Engl J Med 2004;351:1849.

Seizure in a 43-Year-Old Woman

ID/CC: 43-year-old Chinese-American woman with left arm convulsions

HPI: MH was with her daughter in a grocery store when her left arm began to convulse. She asked her daughter to call her husband for help, and he came to find her left arm and leg shaking. He called 911, and she was brought to a community hospital. She was given a phenytoin sodium (Dilantin) load with 1 g IV. She became sleepy and vomited twice and so was paralyzed and intubated. CT scan revealed a small right parietal hemorrhage at the gray-white junction. She was then transferred to the nearest regional academic hospital. There was no noted aura, incontinence, or tongue biting. No report of headache, fever, or weight loss in the prior days to weeks.

PMHx: None

PSHx: None

Meds: None, including no oral contraceptives

All: NKDA

FHx: No history of cancer, clotting disorders

SHx: Married mother of one daughter

Habits: No tobacco, no alcohol, no IVDA or recreational drugs

VS: Temp 98.9°F BP 135/80 HR 78 RR 12 on ventilator

PE: intubated but awake and alert; no visible head trauma, neck supple, no bruits, normal breath sounds, regular cardiac rhythm, no abdominal masses, no rashes or petechiae, no calf tenderness or cords

Neuro: Within the limits of being intubated, neurologic examination is normal, including no papilledema, no focal weakness, and normal reflexes.

Labs/drug screen: Normal chemistry and LFT panel, CBC, and routine coagulation studies. Urinalysis is unremarkable.

THOUGHT QUESTIONS

- What is the differential for the intracranial hemorrhage in this case?
- What studies would help differentiate between the possible diagnoses?

The hemorrhage in this case is atypical for several reasons. The most common cause of intracerebral hemorrhages overall—and particularly in middle-aged people—is chronic HTN. Lesions usually occur in the basal ganglia, thalamus, pons, cerebellum, or deep white matter. The patient has no history of HTN and her lesion is uncharacteristic. It is also atypical for a subcortical lesion to cause seizure, and should raise suspicion of some other process irritating the cortex. Possible etiologies in this case include tumor, vascular malformation, aneurysm rupture, hemorrhagic transformation of ischemic infarct, and venous sinus thrombosis with infarct and hemorrhage.

CT or MRI with angiography is indicated. In order to obtain a rapid image to determine if the hemorrhage has enlarged and to obtain better anatomic detail of intracerebral arteries, it is appropriate to obtain CT with and without contrast to assess for enhancing lesions such as tumor, and CT arteriography to assess for arteriovenous malformation (AVM) or aneurysm. At the same time, many institutions now offer CT venography with good resolution of the cerebral venous system to assess for sinus or cortical vein thrombosis. MRI with diffusion-weighted imaging is more sensitive for infarction, and MRI with and without gadolinium is more sensitive for small metastatic tumors. MRV is similar in sensitivity to CT venography for detecting thrombosis in the cerebral venous system; however, MRA is not as sensitive as computed tomography angiography (CTA) for intracerebral AVM or aneurysm. Conventional angiography is the gold standard for these vascular malformations, but is invasive and more time-consuming and thus not the first choice in the acute setting. Conventional angiography would be indicated only if CT and MRI techniques were unrevealing.

CASE CONTINUED

CT with and without contrast, as well as CTA and CT venography, is obtained. This reveals that the hemorrhage is stable in size without signs of mass effect and shows no evidence of AVM, aneurysm, or underlying tumor. CT venography is significant for loss of contrast filling in the superior sagittal sinus, with engorgement of a right parietal cortical vein overlying the area of hemorrhage, consistent with sinus thrombosis.

THOUGHT QUESTIONS

- What are the causes of cerebral sinus thrombosis?
- What further work-up is indicated?
- What is the standard treatment of cerebral sinus thrombosis?

Cerebral sinus thrombosis is more common in young adults and children. Approximately 75% of patients are women. It is thought that most patients have an underlying prothrombotic state with a precipitating factor leading to the sinus thrombosis. Causes of hypercoagulability include pregnancy, use of oral contraceptives, genetic clotting disorders such as Factor V Leiden mutation, and acquired disorders such as antiphospholipid antibody syndrome. Precipitating factors include head trauma, childbirth, jugular vein or neurosurgical instrumentation, or infections such as mastoiditis or otitis. In children, congenital heart disease with chronic hypoxemia can lead to polycythemia with increased viscosity leading to venous stasis and thrombosis.

Further history should be obtained to determine if there is an unidentified personal or family history of clotting as evidenced by frequent miscarriages or deep venous thrombosis. Normal screening studies rule out nephrotic syndrome and polycythemia syndromes. A pregnancy test should be obtained. Laboratory studies for prothrombotic states should be obtained, including tests for antithrombin deficiency, protein C and S deficiency, Factor V Leiden mutation, prothrombin gene mutation, and antiphospholipid antibody syndrome. If these studies are unrevealing, screening for malignancy with CT scan of the chest, abdomen, and pelvis should be considered.

The standard treatment for cerebral sinus thrombosis is anticoagulation with heparin acutely, with conversion to warfarin for at least 6 months, sometimes longer if predisposing factors are found. Despite the frequent occurrence of hemorrhage before the initiation of anticoagulation, the enlargement of hemorrhage or new hemorrhage does not occur. In addition to preventing extension of cerebral sinus thromboses, anticoagulation helps prevent clots from forming elsewhere or leading to embolic events such as pulmonary embolism. In cases of severe thrombosis with increased intracranial pressure and signs of herniation or severe infarction, surgical thrombectomy or endovascular thrombolysis is performed.

 CASE CONTINUED

The patient was started on IV heparin and quickly extubated. Follow-up examination revealed no focal neurologic signs. Dilantin was continued without further seizure activity. MRI with MRV was obtained, which revealed restricted diffusion in the area of the hemorrhage, consistent with venous infarction, and MRV confirmed a flow void in the superior sagittal sinus.

 QUESTIONS

5-1. Which of the following hypercoagulable states is associated with arterial as well as venous thrombosis?
   A. Antiphospholipid antibody syndrome
   B. Factor V Leiden mutation
   C. Protein C deficiency
   D. Prothrombin gene mutation

5-2. What is the most common location of cerebral sinus thrombosis?
   A. Superior sagittal sinus
   B. Straight sinus
   C. Transverse sinuses
   D. Jugular veins

5-3. Which of the following symptoms might you expect in the early stages of cerebral sinus thrombosis?
   A. Headache
   B. Diplopia
   C. Visual impairment
   D. All of the above

5-4. Which of the following predisposes individuals to a venous thrombosis?
   A. Dehydration
   B. Excess green vegetables
   C. Steroids
   D. Aspirin

 ANSWERS

5-1. A. All of the disorders listed cause venous thromboses leading to complications such as deep venous thrombosis and pulmonary embolism. Antiphospholipid antibody syndrome, associated with anticardiolipin and lupus coagulant, causes both venous and arterial thrombosis and is thus a potential source of ischemic strokes, particularly in young patients.

5-2. C. In many cases, more than one sinus or vein is affected. The most common locations, in decreasing order, are transverse sinuses (86%), superior sagittal sinus (62%), straight sinus (18%), cortical veins (17%), and jugular veins (12%).

5-3. D. All of the symptoms listed can be seen with increased intracranial pressure, such as that caused by a blockage in CSF reuptake by cerebral sinus thrombosis. Headache is present in more than 90% of adult patients and is often severe. Diplopia can result from increased pressure on cranial nerve VI, and papilledema can lead to transient visual impairment.

5-4. A. Hypercoagulable states are worsened by anything in the Virchow triad of stasis, hypercoagulability, and endothelial dysfunction. Dehydration leads to vascular stasis and will increase the incidence of clot formation.

 ADDITIONAL SUGGESTED READING

Duchowny M, Harve AS. Pediatric epilepsy syndromes: an update and critical review. Epilepsia 1996;37(Suppl 1):S26.
Shinnar S, O'Dell C, Berg AT. Distribution of epilepsy syndromes in a cohort of children prospectively monitored from the time of their first unprovoked seizure. Epilepsia 1999;40:1378.

Seizures in an 8-Year-Old Girl

ID/CC: 8-year-old girl with two seizures

HPI: RE is an 8-year-old right-handed girl brought in to a pediatric neurologist's office with a history of two seizures. The first episode occurred 1 month prior to presentation, the second 3 weeks later. Both occurred in the early hours of the morning, when the child was asleep. Her father heard some guttural sounds coming from her bedroom, and when he went to check on her, the right side of her face was twitching. She then proceeded to develop generalized tonic-clonic activity. Each episode lasted 45 seconds and stopped. Right after she seemed a little disoriented and had trouble speaking.

PMHx: Normal birth and development, no chronic illnesses

Meds: None

All: None

FHx: The child's mother had febrile seizures as a toddler

SHx: Straight A student in school

PE/Neuro: General and detailed neurologic examination: Normal

THOUGHT QUESTIONS

▪ How will you classify this child's seizure?

▪ What evaluation does she need to arrive at a diagnosis?

Key points in the history and description of the episode help in classification of this child's seizure. Clearly, she had a seizure that initially involved only the right side of her face. As the seizure progressed, her entire body was involved, with rhythmic, clonic jerks. Thus the seizure had a partial or focal onset, but eventually became generalized. This is a partial seizure with secondary generalization. A seizure that starts with bilateral manifestations is a generalized-from-onset seizure (Table 6-1).

TABLE **6-1**   International League Against Epilepsy (ILAE) Classification of Seizures

Partial Seizures *Simple (no loss of consciousness or memory)*	Generalized Seizures *Tonic-clonic*	Unclassified Seizures
1. Sensory	Tonic	
2. Motor	Clonic	
3. Sensory-motor	Atonic	
4. Autonomic (heat, nausea, flushing)	Absence	
5. Psychic (abnormal thoughts or perceptions: e.g., déjà vu)	Myoclonic	
Complex (consciousness/memory impaired)		
1. With or without aura		
2. With or without automatisms		
Secondarily generalized		

A seizure results from abnormal synchronous electrical activity in the brain. It consists of paroxysmal sensory, motor, or behavioral symptoms. Epilepsy is a chronic condition where unprovoked seizures occur repeatedly. In order to classify seizures and the type of epilepsy in a particular patient, the following work-up is required:

(1) Complete history and PE (including a detailed neurologic examination)
(2) Epilepsy risk factors (prior CNS insults/infections/trauma, family history of epilepsy)
(3) EEG findings
(4) Neuroimaging data (MRI scan)

Using this approach, the International League Against Epilepsy (ILAE) recognizes four epilepsy syndromes, based on the type of seizures and etiology of the seizures (Table 6-2).

1. Idiopathic generalized epilepsy
2. Idiopathic localization-related epilepsy
3. Symptomatic generalized epilepsy
4. Symptomatic localization-related epilepsy

TABLE 6-2 ILAE Recognized Epilepsy Syndromes

Idiopathic Localization Related Epilepsy	Symptomatic Localization Related Epilepsy
Partial seizures	Partial seizures
Normal intellect	Gross/subtle cognitive abnormalities
Normal PE	Gross/subtle abnormalities on examination
Positive family history	Variable family history
Normal EEG background	Abnormal EEG background
Focal spikes	Focal spikes
Normal neuroimaging	Abnormal neuroimaging
Good prognosis	Variable prognosis
Idiopathic generalized epilepsy	**Symptomatic generalized epilepsy**
Generalized seizures	Generalized seizures
Normal intellect	Subnormal intellect
Normal PE	Abnormal PE
Positive family history	Variable family history
Normal EEG background	Abnormal EEG background
Bisynchronous (generalized) spikes	Bisynchronous (generalized) spikes
Normal neuroimaging	Abnormal neuroimaging
Good prognosis	Poor prognosis

 CASE CONTINUED

She had an EEG, which shows a focal epileptiform abnormality in the left central-temporal region. Her MRI scan and screening laboratory tests (CBC, electrolytes, etc.) were normal.

 THOUGHT QUESTION

■ What is her epilepsy diagnosis?

This patient is developmentally normal and has a normal neurologic examination. Her only risk factor is a family history of febrile seizures in her mother. Her EEG shows a focal abnormality and she has normal neuroimaging studies. The features of her epilepsy fit the idiopathic localization related epilepsy syndrome (the specific name for her type of epilepsy is benign rolandic epilepsy). Features in her presentation that are typical for benign rolandic epilepsy are: semiology of her seizures, family history, EEG findings, normal examination, and neuroimaging. These children present in mid to late childhood with secondarily generalized seizures that are often nocturnal or in the early hours of the morning. Their seizures are easy to treat with antiepileptic drugs, and usually seizures remit in adolescence.

QUESTIONS

6-1. Febrile seizures differ from childhood epilepsy syndrome by which of the following features?
- A. Occur in children ages 6 months to 5 years
- B. May occur in association with a fever
- C. Duration is typically 5 minutes or shorter
- D. Treatment with anti-epileptic drugs is not indicated

6-2. Which of the following is an example of idiopathic generalized epilepsy?
- A. Absence epilepsy of childhood
- B. Infantile spasms
- C. Posttraumatic epilepsy
- D. Benign rolandic epilepsy
- E. Lennox-Gastaut's syndrome

6-3. Which of the following is the drug of choice for treating absence seizures?
- A. Phenytoin
- B. Gabapentin
- C. Valproic acid
- D. Carbamazepine
- E. Tiagabine

6-4. What is Todd paralysis?
A. Transient weakness of the side involved in the seizure
B. Paralysis of upgaze
C. Neither
D. Both

 ANSWERS

6-1. D. Febrile seizures are fairly common in children 6 months to 5 years old. They usually occur in conjunction with a febrile illness, and the etiology of the fever is outside the CNS. Seizures are typically the generalized tonic-clonic type, and are brief in duration. Febrile seizures presenting as status epilepticus are also known. Treatment with chronic antiepileptic drugs is not recommended.

6-2. A. Absence epilepsy is an idiopathic generalized epilepsy syndrome. Infantile spasms is a descriptive term used for a particular type of generalized seizure, and is most commonly seen in infants with symptomatic generalized epilepsy. Posttraumatic epilepsy is an example of symptomatic localization-related epilepsy. Benign rolandic epilepsy is an example of idiopathic localization-related epilepsy. The child in the case described above is a typical example of this syndrome.

6-3. C. Valproic acid, ethosuximide, and lamotrigine are drugs used to treat absence seizures. The others are commonly used to treat partial seizures.

6-4. A. Todd paralysis is a transient hemiparesis of the side of the body involved in a partial seizure. It is a temporary phenomenon and resolves within hours. Paralysis of upgaze results from lesions in the midbrain; it is not a cortical phenomenon.

 ADDITIONAL SUGGESTED READING

Stam J. Thrombosis of the cerebral veins and sinuses. N Engl J Med 2005;352:1791–1798.

II

Patients Who Present with Involuntary Movements

Tremor in Adulthood

ID/CC: 55-year-old right-handed man presents with a tremor in his right hand.

HPI: Over the last year HT has noticed a worsening tremor in his right hand. His tremor is most noticeable when he is walking or watching television and gets worse when he is nervous. It is not relieved by alcohol and disappears when he is cooking and playing tennis. On neurologic review of systems, Mr. T complains of needing a longer time to get ready for work in the morning, slowing down of his tennis game, and a change in his handwriting. He has not had any recent head injuries or falls.

PMHx: HTN

PSHx: Appendectomy at age 36

Meds: Metoprolol 50 mg two times a day

All: NKDA

SHx: Lifelong nonsmoker, lawyer, married, lives in a rural community

FHx: HTN, HD. No family history of tremor.

Neuro Hx: None

THOUGHT QUESTIONS

- What is a tremor and how can they be subclassified?
- What is your differential diagnosis? (at least three possibilities)
- What signs will you look for on examination to aid in diagnosis?
- What are cardinal and associated features of Parkinson's disease?

A tremor is a rhythmic, oscillating movement caused by synchronous or alternating contractions of antagonist muscles. Tremors can be classified based on their distribution (limb, head, chin, trunk, etc.), frequency (slow, fast), etiology (parkinsonian, cerebellar, etc.), or most commonly, phenomenology (rest or action). Rest tremors are present when the body part is completely supported against gravity (like resting on the lap or table for a hand tremor) and when the muscles are not voluntarily being contracted. Rest tremors disappear or at the very least, diminish significantly when the affected body part is voluntarily being used. Action tremors occur when a body part is voluntarily being used and disappear at rest unless they are very severe. Action tremors can be subclassified into postural tremors (antigravity posture like outstretching the arms), kinetic tremors (during the course of a voluntary movement like the finger-to-nose test) and task- or position-specific tremors (like a vocal tremor when singing only or only while holding a cup).

In this patient the history gives some good clues about the nature of the tremor. Because it disappears when he is playing tennis it points strongly toward a rest tremor. The differential diagnosis of the onset of a chronic asymmetric rest tremor should include Parkinson's disease, past history of neuroleptic exposure, parkinsonism, and Parkinson's plus syndromes.

On examination the type of tremor should be documented. Other important signs for differential diagnosis include posture, gait, and tone. Parkinson's plus syndromes are very rare but carry a much poorer prognosis and often do not respond to treatment. Therefore, signs of dementia, autonomic dysfunction, neuromuscular disease, dystonia, and eye movement abnormalities should be assessed as well.

The five cardinal features of Parkinson's disease are tremor, bradykinesia, rigidity, loss of postural reflexes, and the freezing phenomenon (akinesia). Freezing, postural instability, and bradykinesia are grouped as negative phenomena and are more disabling than tremor and rigidity (the positive phenomena). Unfortunately, the negative symptoms do not respond as well to treatment. Masked facies, micrographia, decreased glabellar reflex, stooped posture, decreased arm swing, and difficulties with pivot turns are all associated features of the disease. Symptoms usually begin asymmetrically or unilaterally, as in this patient. As the disease progresses, the motor symptoms worsen and often become resistant to treatment, autonomic symptoms appear, and cognitive and affective symptoms may develop.

CASE CONTINUED

VS: Temp 98.6°F BP 110/70 HR 76 RR 16. Normal orthostatics

PE: Normal, well-appearing man. No organomegaly.

Neuro: MSE: alert and oriented times 4, MMSE 30/30

CN II–XII: Intact. Normal extraocular eye movements.

**Motor and
coordination:**   Normal bulk and strength throughout. Slowed right hand rapid alternating movements. Cogwheeling in right wrist. Gross, pill-rolling resting tremor in right hand remits with intentional movements.

Reflexes: 2+ throughout. No Babinski signs present.

Sensory: Intact to light touch, pinprick, vibration and temperature throughout.

Gait: Normal posture, stride, speed, and pivot turns. Decreased arm swing on the right. No ataxia, intact tandem gait.

QUESTIONS

7-1. Parkinson's disease is caused by which of the following?
   A. Degeneration of the GABAergic neurons in the putamen
   B. Degeneration of the cholinergic neurons in the nucleus basalis
   C. Degeneration of the dopaminergic neurons in the substantia nigra
   D. Degeneration of the glutamatergic neurons in the subthalamic nucleus
   E. Degeneration of the serotonin neurons in the raphe nucleus

7-2. What is the incidence of dementia in Parkinson's disease?
   A. 5% to 10%
   B. 10% to 30%
   C. 25% to 50%
   D. 40% to 65%
   E. Greater than 65%

7-3. Which of the following medications is used frequently to treat Parkinson's disease?
A. Topamax (topiramate)
B. Sinemet (carbidopa/levodopa)
C. Alcohol
D. β-blockers (atenolol)
E. Reserpine

7-4. What is the pathologic hallmark of Parkinson's disease?
A. Hirano bodies
B. Pick bodies
C. Negri bodies
D. Lewy bodies
E. Senile plaques

 ANSWERS

7-1. C. Parkinson's disease is caused by the degeneration of the dopaminergic neurons in the substantia nigra. This leads to dysfunction in the nigrostriatal pathways and upsets the normal balance between the dopaminergic-cholinergic systems. Degeneration of the GABAergic neurons in the putamen is the hallmark of Huntington's disease. Degeneration of the cholinergic neurons in the nucleus basalis occurs in Alzheimer's disease. Damage to the glutamatergic neurons in the subthalamic nucleus leads to hemiballismus and is usually caused by a stroke.

7-2. B. Common cognitive and affective symptoms associated with Parkinson's disease are depression, dementia, and bradyphrenia (slowness of thinking). While the estimates of the incidence of dementia in Parkinson's disease vary widely, largely because of tertiary care center biased studies and difficulty in excluding Parkinson-plus diseased patients from estimates, somewhere between 10% to 30% of patients with Parkinson's disease will develop a true global dementia late in their disease course. Early appearance of dementia out of proportion to motor findings should prompt a thorough evaluation for Parkinson's plus syndromes.

7-3. D. Sinemet is still the best symptomatic treatment available for Parkinson's disease but it has many side effects at higher doses. Dopamine agonists also provide some symptomatic relief and are often used in combination with Sinemet. Monoamine oxidase type B (MAO-B) inhibitors provide some symptomatic relief and may have a long-term protective effect. β-blockers are used to treat essential and physiologic tremors.

7-4. D. The pathologic hallmark of Parkinson's disease is Lewy bodies. Lewy bodies are round, intracytoplasmic inclusions found in the pigmented neurons of the substantia nigra. Hirano bodies are associated with Alzheimer's disease and extracellular. Negri bodies are associated with rabies. Pick bodies are basophilic cytoplasmic inclusions found in the cortex.

 ADDITIONAL SUGGESTED READING

Cohen O, Pullman S, Jurewicz E, et al. Rest tremor in patients with essential tremor: prevalence, clinical correlates, and electrophysiologic characteristics. Arch Neurol 2003;60:405.

Louis ED, Ford B, Frucht S, et al. Risk of tremor and impairment from tremor in relatives of patients with essential tremor: a community-based family study. Ann Neurol 2001;49:761.

Child with Involuntary Movements

ID/CC: 10-year-old boy with involuntary movements

HPI: SC is a 10-year-old right-handed male referred for evaluation of involuntary movements. The boy was in his usual state of health 2 to 3 weeks ago, when he first developed difficulty walking. His mother described a lurching quality to his gait. Gradually over time his walking got worse, and he began falling down while walking. Over the last few days, his upper extremities have developed intermittent writhing movements, making it progressively difficult to eat or write. In fact the boy's teachers have noticed a clear change in handwriting, and that he has difficulty sitting still and "keeping his hands to himself." The movements occur intermittently throughout the day, increase when he is tired, will reduce if he focuses intently upon them, and remits during sleep.

PMHx: Normal birth and development. History of chronic sinusitis, and history of URI with sore throat 6 weeks ago

PSHx: Negative

Meds: Claritin occasionally for seasonal allergies

All: NKDA

FHx: Noncontributory

SHx: One of four siblings. Mother and father work outside the house.

PE: Gen: VS normal. No dysmorphic features. Occasional cervical lymph node palpable. Remainder of general examination normal.

Neuro: Mental status: normal orientation and attention

Speech: Dysarthric

CN II–XII: Intact

Motor
examination: Tone: normal. Strength 5/5 in right upper and lower extremities, 4/5 in left upper and lower extremities.

Reflexes: Normal. Frequent involuntary jerking is seen in SC's extremities, involving his upper and lower extremities, trunk, and face. His left arm, leg, and face are more affected than the right. He is unable to stand because of constant involuntary movements and unable to eat because of the jerking and lurching movements of his arms. In fact he can hardly lie still from all these movements. When observed during sleep, the movements cease.

THOUGHT QUESTIONS

- How will you characterize these movements?
- What work-up will you do to establish a diagnosis and etiology?

Involuntary motor phenomena include movement disorders stemming from basal ganglia pathology, myoclonus, and seizures.

Chorea is an involuntary movement that consists of brief, sudden irregular, purposeless jerking movements of the limbs, trunk, face, or combination thereof. The movements may involve one or both sides of the body, are often worse with stress and when attention is drawn to them, and remit in sleep. There is inability to maintain sustained muscle contraction, leading to a waxing and waning quality to the patient's hand grip (milk-maid grip), or darting, in-and-out movements on protrusion of the tongue (Jack-in-the-box tongue).

Athetosis is an involuntary movement with slow, writhing movements of larger amplitude. The movements tend to affect more distal muscles than what is seen with chorea, but distinction between chorea and athetosis can be difficult.

Ballismus is a large amplitude involuntary movement, with a flinging (flailing) quality to it. It usually involves one limb/side of the body, and can be nearly continuous when awake. This involuntary movement also ceases during sleep.

Dystonia is an involuntary movement with slow, sustained movements with a twisting or contorting quality to them. These movements may involve limited groups of muscles, one limb, one half of the body, or they may be generalized. They may be precipitated by specific movements.

Tics are brief, abrupt, stereotyped movements that occur at regular or irregular intervals. They consist of movements such as shoulder shrugging, eye blinking, and so on. There is often an urge for an individual to move, and this can be suppressed to some extent. They may exhibit a waxing and waning pattern over time (during the day or over several days or weeks). They are often exacerbated by stress and relieved by distraction.

Myoclonus is a movement disorder with sudden, brisk, lightning-like contraction of a muscle or group of muscles. The movements may be repetitive, and at times forceful.

A seizure is a paroxysmal alteration of sensory, motor, or behavioral function that results from an abnormal, hypersynchronous electrical discharge from the cerebral cortex.

In the above case, the near-constant presence of the movements and their disappearance during sleep is characteristic of a movement disorder. Based on their description, the most likely diagnosis is chorea or athetosis.

Laboratory work-up is directed at establishing the etiology of the chorea. Table 8-1 summarizes conditions associated with chorea.

TABLE 8-1 Causes of Chorea

Hereditary Conditions	**Vascular**	**Drugs**
Huntington's disease	Basal ganglia stroke/ hemorrhage	Neuroleptics
Wilson's disease		Antiparkinsonian drugs
Hallervorden-Spatz's disease		Antiepileptic drugs: phenytoin, carbamazepine
Infectious/immunologic	**Metabolic/endocrine**	**Miscellaneous**
Sydenham chorea (poststreptococcal)	Pregnancy (chorea gravidarum)	Kernicterus
Viral encephalitis	Hyperthyroidism	Aminoacidopathies
Systemic lupus erythematosus	Hepatic/renal encephalopathy	
Sarcoidosis		

CASE CONTINUED

Lab: CBC: WNL, electrolytes, glucose, LFTs: WNL. ESR: 35 mm. ANA: negative. ASO titer: 1:1260 (elevated). Serum copper and ceruloplasmin levels: WNL. T4 and TSH: WNL

Imaging: MRI brain: Increased T2 signal in both basal ganglia (right greater than left). Trinucleotide repeats are sent, and results are pending.

THOUGHT QUESTION

- How does this work-up assist in the diagnosis?

The lack of fever or other prodrome makes a viral encephalitis unlikely. His normal ANA, LFTs, copper and ceruloplasmin levels rule out conditions like systemic lupus erythematosus, Wilson's disease, or other hepatic disorders. Thyroid dysfunction is not likely. The elevated ESR and ASO titer are diagnostic of Sydenham's chorea (St. Vitus, dance).

QUESTIONS

8-1. Sydenham's chorea is a sequel of:
A. Herpes simplex infection
B. Streptococcal infection
C. An inborn error of metabolism
D. Idiopathic
E. Malignancy

8-2. Which of the following drugs can produce a movement disorder?
A. Acetaminophen
B. Digitalis
C. Haloperidol
D. Propranolol
E. Simvastatin

8-3. Tics are part of the following disorder:
A. Lennox-Gastaut's syndrome
B. Landau-Kleffner's syndrome
C. Gilles de la Tourette's syndrome
D. Lambert-Eaton's syndrome
E. Guillain Barré's syndrome

8-4. In a patient with hemiballismus, what is the location of the lesion?
A. Subthalamic nucleus
B. Red nucleus
C. Supraoptic nucleus
D. Hypothalamus
E. Thalamus

ANSWERS

8-1. B. Sydenham's chorea (St. Vitus' dance) is an immune-mediated postinfectious cause of chorea. It occurs as a sequel of infection with Group A β-hemolytic streptococcus. It is most common between ages 5 and 25 years. Clinical manifestations include an acute or subacute onset of chorea, which may be asymmetric in its severity. Mild weakness in muscle strength is not unusual. Characteristically, antibodies to streptococcal antigens are elevated, indicating prior infection. T2 signal changes in the basal ganglia have been described. The chorea can be treated with benzodiazepines, valproate, or haloperidol. Long-term penicillin treatment is indicated for preventing further streptococcal infections.

8-2. C. Haloperidol and other neuroleptic medications can produce movement disorders such as chorea or tardive dyskinesia. Acetaminophen and digitalis do not produce movement disorders. Propranolol is used in the treatment of essential tremor, another movement disorder.

8-3. C. Tics are part of Gilles de la Tourette's syndrome. Lennox-Gastaut is a condition with seizures, mental retardation, and characteristic EEG findings. Landau-Kleffner is a rare syndrome with language regression, autistic behavior, and seizures.

8-4. A. Lesions in the subthalamic nucleus produce ballismus (or hemiballismus). The most common etiology for subthalamic nucleus lesions is stroke. Other causes include infection, demyelinating diseases, and tumor.

ADDITIONAL SUGGESTED READING

Cardoso F, Camargos S. Juvenile parkinsonism: a heterogeneous
    entity. Eur J Neurol 2000;7:467.
Jankovic J. Tourette's syndrome. N Engl J Med 2001;345:1184.

Fluctuating Tremor in an Adult

 ID/CC: 51-year-old right-handed man presents with a fluctuating tremor in his right hand.

HPI: Over the last 2 years HC has noticed a worsening tremor in his right hand. He first noticed when trying to sign a witnessed legal document 10 years ago. Over the last 2 years he has noticed it daily and now he has difficulty drinking a cup of coffee without spilling. It is not present at rest. Once an excellent public speaker, his wife reports that his voice has become tremulous during several recent public speeches.

PMHx: None

PSHx: None

Meds: None

All: NKDA

SHx: Minister, married. Moderate alcohol consumption, nonsmoker. No history of illicit drug use.

FHx: Mother had lifelong tremors in her hands and eventually tremors of her head and trunk. She never sought medical attention for the tremors.

Neuro Hx: None. No history of neuroleptic exposure.

THOUGHT QUESTIONS

- What is your differential diagnosis? (at least three possibilities)
- What signs will you look for on examination and what laboratory tests will you order to aid in diagnosis?

■ Discuss the clinical findings, etiology, and disease course in adult-onset Huntington's disease.

Tremors fall into three broad categories: action, resting, and intention tremor. An action tremor is one that is associated with a posture or appears only with activity and disappears with rest, as in this man. The differential diagnosis of an action tremor is (1) essential (or familial) tremor, (2) tremor associated with pheochromocytoma, amphetamines, lithium, corticosteroids, β-agonists, and hyperthyroidism, and rarely, (3) Wilson's disease, and (4) atypical Huntington's disease. Action tremors are frequently worse when the patient is nervous and improve with alcohol. Wilson's disease is a rare, autosomal recessive disorder of copper metabolism that usually presents in adolescence or early adulthood with psychiatric disturbances often dominating the clinical picture.

Physical and laboratory examination should (1) define the type of tremor; (2) look for signs of pheochromocytoma and hyperthyroidism including TFTs; (3) look for signs of Wilson's disease such as Kayser-Fleischer rings (copper deposition in the Descemet's membrane of the cornea), hepatitis, liver cirrhosis, renal dysfunction, hypersplenism, and hemolytic anemia; and (4) look for movement abnormalities in other body parts.

Huntington's disease is a hereditary, progressive movement disorder that typically causes chorea, psychiatric disturbances, dementia, and, as the disease progresses, parkinsonism (decreased arm swing, dystonias, and bradykinesia). Early in the disease course the chorea may not be evident and the abnormal movements may simply be described as clumsiness, twitching, jerking, or incoordination. The disease may present with psychiatric symptoms of depression, schizophreniform disorder, paranoid psychosis, or just personality changes. Clinical examination usually reveals chorea and impersistence of sustained motor movements such as handgrip or tongue protrusion (i.e., the patient is unable to keep his tongue stretched out and involuntarily retracts it). Chorea is defined as involuntary, abrupt, rapid, irregular, unsustained movements that flow randomly from one body part to another. Movement abnormalities are frequently defined not only by the limbs but also by the joints that they involve. Oculomotor abnormalities are another clinical hallmark of Huntington's disease. These include saccadic pursuit, convergence paresis, and impersistence of gaze.

Rarely, adult-onset Huntington's disease can present with predominantly parkinsonian features without chorea. Bradykinesia, rigidity, action tremor, and myoclonus are prominent in these patients. This form of Huntington's disease (the Westphal variant) is most frequently seen in the juvenile-onset cases of Huntington's disease (younger than 20 years old).

Huntington's disease is caused by a CAG trinucleotide repeat expansion on the short arm of chromosome 4. Normal individuals have fewer than 30 of these repeats whereas Huntington's disease patients have more than 40 and juvenile-onset Huntington's disease is associated with 50 or more repeats. The disease is inherited in an autosomal dominant fashion and is usually worse when transmitted from paternal lineage. The disease results in marked atrophy of the caudate and putamen and to a lesser extent, global cerebral atrophy. Neurons from multiple neurotransmitter systems (most markedly gamma-aminobutyric acid [GABA] and acetylcholine) are affected, making even symptomatic treatment difficult with only a relative sparing of neuropeptide Y-somatostatin neurons.

 CASE CONTINUED

VS: Temp 98.6°F BP 110/70 HR 76 RR 16

PE: Gen: Normal, well-appearing man. No Kaiser-Fleischer rings. No hepatomegaly.

Neuro: MSE: Fully oriented. MMSE: 30/30. Mood is good. Affect is appropriate. Thought content is clear and coherent.

CN II–XII: Intact.

Motor: 5/5 strength throughout with normal bulk and tone. No cogwheeling is present

Reflexes: 2+ throughout. No Babinski signs present bilaterally

Sensory: Intact to light touch, pinprick, vibration, and temperature throughout

Coordination: Fine, regular tremor in both arms when outstretched, more pronounced on the right. Worsens significantly when asked to pour water into a cup. Not present at rest. No dysmetria. No chorea or motor impersistence. No rigidity or akinesia.

Gait: Normal, no ataxia

Labs: TSH and free T4 WNL

QUESTIONS

9-1. What is the most likely diagnosis?
   A. Drug-induced
   B. Physiologic tremor ("stage fright")
   C. Essential tremor
   D. Parkinson's disease
   E. Stroke

9-2. Which of the following is an appropriate treatment option?
   A. Sinemet
   B. Propranolol
   C. Amantadine
   D. Trihexyphenidyl
   E. Selegiline

9-3. Which of the following may improve his tremor?
   A. Heat
   B. Cheese
   C. Fear
   D. Caffeine
   E. Alcohol

9-4. If initial medical therapy does not provide benefit, which of the following therapeutic options has shown efficacy in patients with essential tremor?
   A. Pallidotomy
   B. Frontal lobotomy
   C. Acupuncture
   D. Fish oil
   E. Transcranial magnetic stimulation

ANSWERS

9-1. C. Essential tremor is the most likely diagnosis given his PE findings, the duration of his tremor, and now the appearance of an episodic vocal tremor. He is not taking any drugs associated with action tremors, he has a family history of tremors, and the tremor occurs even in private settings when he is not nervous.

9-2. C. Most patients with essential tremor respond well to primidone, propranolol, or diazepam, although diazepam is usually used only for patients with intermittent tremors, such as this patient had 10 years ago, or in those patients who do not respond or cannot tolerate primidone and propranolol. Sinemet use is not helpful.

9-3. E. Worsening of symptoms with heat is typical in multiple sclerosis patients. As with any action tremor, his is likely to be made worse by caffeine and nervousness. A diagnostic clue to essential tremor is that patients often report several hours of relief after ingesting low doses of alcohol.

9-4. D. While most people with essential tremor never seek medical attention for their tremor, in the 10% that do, it often interferes with daily function. In this man it is quite likely that it will become disabling, most likely interfering with his ability to feed himself. More than 60% of patients with essential tremor experience excellent symptomatic relief with primidone or propranolol only. Should he not respond to either of these treatments there are potential surgical options including deep-brain stimulation and pallidotomy. Frontal lobotomy is not indicated in this setting.

 ADDITIONAL SUGGESTED READINGS

Brewer GJ, Fink JK, Hedera P. Diagnosis and treatment of Wilson's disease. Semin Neurol 1999;19:261.
Martin JB. Mechanisms of disease: molecular basis of the neurodegenerative disorders. N Engl J Med 1999;340:1970–1980.

CASE **10**

Infant with Episodic Body Jerking

ID/CC: 7-month-old infant with sudden jerking of the body.

HPI: TS is a 7-month-old male who was seen by his pediatrician for episodes of body jerking. These were described as sudden onset flexion of arms and legs, drawing up of legs on the abdomen, slight flexion of the neck, followed by a distressed cry. An individual episode lasted a few seconds. They occurred singly or in clusters, most frequent when the child was falling asleep or awakening. The episodes began 2 months ago. Initially they were thought to be infant colic, and the parents tried OTC simethicone, with no relief. The episodes had gradually increased in frequency to several per day over the last 2 months.

PMHx: Normal labor and delivery, uneventful pregnancy

Meds: None

All: None

FHx: Noncontributory

SHx: Only child

THOUGHT QUESTIONS

■ What is your differential diagnosis?

■ What additional history will assist in making a diagnosis?

The differential diagnosis for paroxysmal events such as these includes seizures, benign sleep myoclonus, dystonia, hyperexplexia, and Sandifer's syndrome.

The episodes described by the parents are paroxysmal, and do not bear any relationship to the infant's feeding times. The lack of history of vomiting or failure to thrive makes Sandifer's syndrome (extensor posturing related to gastroesophageal reflux) unlikely. The infant's movements are not triggered by tactile stimulation, common in hyperexplexia.

The history of developmental delay is important. Presence of developmental delay makes benign infantile myoclonus unlikely. An EEG will also help exclude this from the differential diagnosis.

The paroxysmal nature of the episodes, clustering of spells, and a tendency to occur around times of transition from wakefulness to sleep (and vice versa) are all highly suggestive that these are seizures. The sudden flexion of the extremities, brief duration, and distressed cry that occurs with the clusters are all features consistent with infantile spasms.

Infantile spasms are generalized tonic seizures that occur in children younger than 12 months of age. Their peak incidence is between the ages 3 to 8 months. Clinically, three types of spasms are identified. Flexor type ("Salaam attacks") consist of sudden adduction of the arms and flexion of the head, trunk, and hips. Extensor spasms involve truncal extension, while mixed-type spasms show features of both. They commonly occur in clusters, and may be followed by a distressed cry.

The EEG in infantile spasms shows a characteristic pattern of a high amplitude slow background with multifocal spike wave discharges, termed hypsarrhythmia.

Infantile spasms can be classified as symptomatic or cryptogenic (idiopathic). Symptomatic infantile spasms are those where an etiology is identified for the spasms. Cryptogenic are those where an etiology is presumed but not identified. Developmental outcome is better in children with idiopathic or cryptogenic infantile spasms than in those with symptomatic infantile spasms. Table 10-1 lists some etiologies.

Further history and attention to specific aspects of the examination will assist in identifying the etiology of the infantile spasms. Key points to elucidate on history and exam include: developmental

TABLE **10-1** Infantile Spasms

Idiopathic (Cryptogenic)	Symptomatic
Hypoxic-ischemic encephalopathy	
Tuberous sclerosis	
Aicardi's syndrome	
Cerebral dysgenesis (e.g., lissencephaly)	
Metabolic diseases (e.g., nonketotic hyperglycinemia)	
CNS infections	

history, particularly developmental regression, a detailed skin examination (with a Wood lamp if necessary), family history of neurologic disorders, measurement of head circumference.

 CASE CONTINUED

On further history, the child is developmentally delayed. He began smiling at 6 weeks of age, and was cooing and reaching out for objects between 4 and 5 months of age. He had just begun sitting without support, and was scooting forward on his abdomen. In the past two months, his reaching out has stopped, and his cooing is less frequent. He seems quiet and makes less eye contact than before.

PE: Gen: Weight: 7.6 kg (25th percentile), OFC 41 cm (<5th percentile). CV: 2/6 murmur at left sternal border, Lungs: Clear, Abdomen: No hepatosplenomegaly (HSM). Skin: Hypopigmented macules on back.

Neuro: Alert, vocalized cranial nerve examination normal. Hypotonic extremities and trunk. Moved all extremities equally. DTRS: Plantars: extensor bilaterally.

 THOUGHT QUESTION

■ How does this information shape the differential diagnosis?

The presence of developmental delay makes it unlikely that this child has "idiopathic" or cryptogenic infantile spasms. His normal birth and perinatal history make hypoxic-ischemic encephalopathy less likely. Aicardi's syndrome is an X-linked disorder seen in females. He is microcephalic, which also implies a symptomatic process. The cutaneous lesions, i.e., the hypopigmented macules, are characteristic of tuberous sclerosis.

 QUESTIONS

10-1. Which of the following cutaneous lesions is seen in tuberous sclerosis?
   A. Shagreen patch
   B. Axillary freckles
   C. Port-wine hemangioma
   D. Nevus flammeus

10-2. The following drugs are used in the treatment of infantile spasms:
   A. adrenocorticotropic hormone (ACTH)
   B. Clonazepam
   C. Neither
   D. Both

10-3. What constitutes West's syndrome?
   A. Infantile spasms, tuberous sclerosis, hypsarrhythmia
   B. Infantile spasms, developmental delay, hypsarrhythmia
   C. Infantile spasms, developmental delay, cortical dysplasia
   D. Infantile spasms, café-au-lait spots, developmental delay

10-4. Which of the syndromes is seen in women and is characterized by choreiform movements, gait difficulties, and language difficulty?
   A. Neurofibromatosis
   B. Ataxia-telangiectasia
   C. Sturge-Weber's syndrome
   D. Rett's syndrome

 ANSWERS

10-1. A. Tuberous sclerosis is a condition with multisystem involvement. Cutaneous manifestations are common and often key in the diagnosis. Hypopigmented macules on the skin are the most common. These may have a "confetti-like" appearance, a leaf-like configuration (called Ashleaf macules), or look like a fingerprint.

Erythematous, "acne-like" papules on the face are called adenoma sebaceum. A rough patch on the lumbosacral area called Shagreen patch may be seen; this is also a cutaneous hamartoma. Fibromas that occur under the nails are termed subungual fibromas. Hyperpigmented skin macules may also occur in tuberous sclerosis, although less commonly. Seizures and varying degrees of mental retardation are the most common CNS manifestation. Axillary freckles are characteristic of neurofibromatosis 1. Port-wine hemangiomas of the face are seen in Sturge-Weber's syndrome.

10-2. D. Drugs used in the treatment of infantile spasms regardless of etiology include ACTH, clonazepam, and valproic acid. Infantile spasms due to tuberous sclerosis respond very well to vigabatrin, an antiepileptic drug, currently not available in the United States. Other medications such as topiramate have also been used to treat infantile spasms.

10-3. B. West's syndrome is a triad of infantile spasms, developmental delay, and hypsarrhythmia on the EEG. It does not imply any specific etiology. It was described by Dr. West in his son, in 1841, in an eloquent letter published in the Lancet.

10-4. D. Tuberous sclerosis, neurofibromatosis, and ataxia-telangiectasia are neurocutaneous syndromes. These disorders have characteristic cutaneous markers and characteristic CNS manifestations (Table 10-2). Rett's syndrome is a disorder that affects females, and is characterized by acquired microcephaly, loss of purposeful hand function, hand-wringing movements, a characteristic gait, and loss of language skills. It is a progressive condition.

TABLE **10-2**   Summary of Findings in Neurocutaneous Disorders

Disorder	Cutaneous Signs	CNS Findings
Neurofibromatosis	Café-au-lait spots Axillary freckling Cutaneous neurofibromas	Gliomas, fibromas, other CNS tumors
Sturge-Weber's syndrome	Port wine stain (face)	Seizures, pial venous angioma
Ataxia-telangiectasia	Skin telangiectasia	Choreoathetosis, developmental delay, immune deficiency, lymphoreticular malignancy

ADDITIONAL SUGGESTED READING

de Menezes MA, Rho JM. Clinical and electrographic features of epileptic spasms persisting beyond the second year of life. Epilepsia 2002;43:623.

Gaily E, Liukkonen E, Paetau R, et al. Infantile spasms: diagnosis and assessment of treatment response by video-EEG. Dev Med Child Neurol 2001;43:65.

III

Patients Who Present with a Headache

"Worst Headache of My Life"

ID/CC: 47-year-old woman with complaint of the worst headache of her life.

HPI: While at work, WH developed a sudden severe headache she described as "the worst headache of my life." Minutes later she developed nausea and recurrent episodes of vomiting. She took a Tylenol without relief. Approximately 30 minutes later she asked a coworker to take her to the ER.

PMHx: Hx of hypothyroidism

PSHx: Appendectomy

Meds: Synthroid

All: NKDA

FHx: No family history of cerebral aneurysms

SHx: Married with two children. She works as a software engineer.

Habits: No tobacco, two glasses of wine per night, occasional marijuana use.

VS: Temp 99°F, BP 160/58 HR 87, RR 10

PE/Neuro: The patient is anxious, but in no acute distress. She is awake, alert, and oriented times 3. PERRLA 3 mm to 2 mm bilaterally. There is no meningismus. CN II–XII are intact. There were no focal neurologic deficits detected.

Labs: Hematocrit, 32.9; Platelet, 117; INR, 1.0; PT, 11.1; PTT, 27.8

ECG: Normal sinus rhythm

THOUGHT QUESTIONS

- What is the patient's differential diagnosis?
- Should the head CT be negative, how does that change your differential diagnosis?
- Should the head CT be negative, what additional diagnostic test would you obtain?

WH's history and PE support a differential diagnosis that includes migraine headache and headache secondary to SAH from an aneurysmal rupture. Other conditions in the differential diagnosis include an intracranial space occupying lesion and meningitis. The sudden onset of the headache, especially in a patient without antecedent history of chronic headaches makes migraine (and chronic headache disorders) less likely. A normal neurologic examination and acute presentation of headache preclude a diagnosis of an intracranial tumor. Headache as an isolated symptom is an uncommon presentation of meningitis.

The complaint of "the worst headache of my life" is classic for a subarachnoid hemorrhage, especially when associated with N&V. This is SAH secondary to aneurysmal rupture.

A head CT may help in differentiating between the two entities. The presence of subarachnoid blood would support the diagnosis of SAH versus migraine headache. A negative head CT does not exclude a diagnosis of SAH. Should the head CT be negative, the next step would be to obtain a LP to evaluate the CSF. (See answer to questions below for details regarding the composition of CSF in the setting of SAH.)

CASE CONTINUED

Noncontrast head CT: A moderate amount subarachnoid hemorrhage within the interhemispheric fissure. There is no associated parenchymal hemorrhage or intraventricular hemorrhage. There is no hydrocephalus.

Four-vessel cerebral angiogram: A saccular anterior communicating artery aneurysm is identified.

The patient remained awake and alert. She underwent craniotomy for clipping of cerebral aneurysm. The procedure was successful. She awoke without neurologic deficit and was transferred to the ICU postoperatively.

QUESTIONS

11-1. Which of the following is the most common source of SAH?
- A. Arteriovenous malformations
- B. Rupture of intracranial aneurysm
- C. Trauma
- D. Vasculitis
- E. Amyloid angiopathy

11-2. Which of the following CSF findings is inconsistent with SAH?
- A. Xanthochromia
- B. Elevated protein
- C. Elevated opening pressure on LP
- D. Elevated WBCs
- E. Clear supernatant

11-3. Which of the following is a complication of SAH?
- A. Hypoglycemia
- B. Hypokalemia
- C. Demyelination
- D. Vasospasm
- E. Vasculitis

11-4. What is the patient's Hunt and Hess grade on admission?
- A. Grade 1
- B. Grade 2
- C. Grade 3
- D. Grade 4
- E. Grade 5

ANSWERS

11-1. C. Trauma is the most common cause of SAH. Rupture of intracranial aneurysm is the most common cause of nontraumatic spontaneous SAH. Other causes of spontaneous SAH include arteriovenous malformations (AVMs), vasculitides, carotid artery dissection, and unknown etiology. Identified risk factors for non-traumatic SAH include HTN, oral contraceptive pills, and cigarette smoking. Ten percent to fifteen percent of patients who have experienced a SAH secondary to aneurysmal rupture die prior to receiving medical care. There is another 10% mortality rate from SAH within the first few days. The overall mortality rate increases to 50% to 60% within the first 30 days.

11-2. B. A clear supernatant is not consistent with CSF from a patient who has suffered a SAH. Such a patient usually has xanthochromia. The other findings of increased opening pressure and increased WBC are also consistent with SAH.

11-3. D. All of the above are known complications of aneurysmal SAH. Cerebral ischemia results from associated cerebral vasospasm. Hydrocephalus results from decreased absorptive capacity of the ventricles resulting from the presence of subarachnoid blood. Cardiac abnormalities also occur in the setting of SAH.

11-4. A. The Hunt and Hess Grading scale is one of several grading scales for SAH. The grades range from 1 to 5. Grade 1 describes an asymptomatic patient or a patient with mild headache and slight nuchal rigidity. Grade 2 describes a patient with CN palsy, moderate to severe headache and nuchal rigidity. Grade 3 involves mild focal deficit, lethargy, or confusion. Grades 4 and 5 are the most severe of the grades. Grade 4 describes a patient with stupor, moderate to severe hemiparesis, and early decerebrate rigidity. Grade 5 involves deep coma, decerebrate rigidity, and a moribund appearance. The clinical significance of this grading scale is that it correlates with neurologic outcome. The lower the grade on the scale, the better is the neurologic outcome of the patient.

 ADDITIONAL SUGGESTED READING

Edlow JA, Caplan LR. Primary care: avoiding pitfalls in the diagnosis of subarachnoid hemorrhage. N Engl J Med 2000;342:29–36.

Molyneux A. International Subarachnoid Aneurysm Trial (ISAT) of neurosurgical clipping versus endovascular coiling in 2143 patients with ruptured intracranial aneurysms: a randomised trial. Lancet 2002;360:1267.

Headache and Confusion

ID/CC: 63-year-old man with headache, progressive confusion, nausea, and vomiting.

HPI: HS awoke with a diffuse throbbing headache. He was noted by his wife to be confused, which worsened over the course of the day. He went to bed to "sleep it off" in the afternoon, and when his wife returned she was unable to arouse him and so called 911. She denies any recent head trauma, fevers, or ingestions. The patient was unresponsive to the emergency medical technician (EMT), so was intubated in the field without paralytic agents.

PMHx: HTN, atrial fibrillation, diabetes

PSHx: Appendectomy

Meds: Atenolol, warfarin, lisinopril, insulin

All: PCN → rash

FHx: No history of intracranial tumors, aneurysms, or arteriovenous malformations (AVMs)

SHx: Retired taxi driver, married with two children

Habits: 1/2 PPD tobacco, former heavy alcohol, no IVDA or recreational drugs

VS: Temp 99.5°F   BP 210/100   HR 85   RR 12 on ventilator

PE: Intubated, eyes closed. No head trauma, neck supple, no bruits, clear breath sounds, irregular cardiac rhythm, benign abdomen, no petechiae or rash.

Neuro: Eyes closed, no eye opening to voice but opens eyes to painful stimulus; mumbles unintelligible sounds; pupils equal and reactive; blink to threat bilaterally; EOMI to doll's maneuver; corneal reflexes intact to saline drops; gag intact to endotracheal tube (ETT) manipulation; withdraws from painful stimuli in all four extremities; toes upgoing bilaterally.

Labs/drug screen: Screening labs are notable for glucose of 200, normal CBC, and elevated INR at 3.5.

Imaging: Noncontrast CT scan of the head reveals left thalamic hemorrhage measuring 4 cm × 7 cm × 5 cm, with extension into the left lateral ventricle (Fig. 12-1).

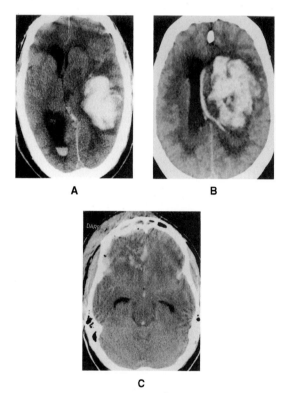

A   **B**

C

FIGURE **12-1** The large hemorrhages into the hemisphere (**A, B**) have resulted in enlargement of the ventricles, a midline shift, and, in the case of A, a small amount of blood in the posterior horn of the lateral ventricle. Hemorrhage into the parenchyma and in the ventricular system may also result from trauma, as in example (**C**), where blood is seen in the frontal lobe and in the third ventricle and cerebral aqueduct. (*From Haines, Duane E. Neuroanatomy: An Atlas of Structures, Sections, and Systems, 6th Ed. Philadelphia: Lippincott, Williams & Wilkins, 2004.*)

THOUGHT QUESTIONS

■ What is the most likely cause of the hemorrhage?

■ What immediate steps should be taken?

HS has several risk factors for intracerebral hemorrhage (ICH). The most common cause of ICH is chronic HTN, which is responsible for up to 75% of ICH. Another important factor in ICH is anticoagulation, and this patient's use of warfarin with INR of 3.5 is likely a contributing factor. Heavy alcohol use is another independent risk factor that could have contributed in this case. Other etiologies include amyloid angiopathy (more common in patients older than the age of 70 years), primary or metastatic brain tumors, and hemorrhagic transformation of prior infarction. Vascular malformations and aneurysms are more common causes in younger populations. ICH in these populations would dictate angiography to assess for vascular malformations or aneurysm as a source.

Several steps can be taken in the acute setting to help prevent extension of the hemorrhage and to help reduce damage secondary to the ICH. Coagulopathies should be corrected immediately. Warfarin can be reversed with IV vitamin K and fresh frozen plasma (FFP). Heparin can be reversed with protamine. Recent studies suggest that recombinant activated factor VII given within 4 hours can decrease growth and reduce mortality, but merits further investigation. The degree of BP control is a debated issue, but most agree that modest control to systolic BP <180 mm Hg is advantageous. Often an arterial line is placed for continuous BP monitoring. If there are signs of imminent herniation on examination or radiographic studies, neurosurgical decompression is a consideration. In this case, the INR of 3.5 and lack of brainstem deficits on examination dictate medical management for the time being. Supportive care is also important, including airway control with mechanical ventilation, monitoring for cardiac ischemia that can accompany ICH, and tight glucose control, which has been shown to reduce secondary cerebral damage. Anti-epileptic medication is not indicated as the patient has not had a seizure and the ICH is not located near the cortex.

CASE CONTINUED

After IV vitamin K and FFP, the INR corrects to 1.3. An arterial line is placed and labetalol is used to bring the BP down below 180 mm Hg. The patient remains intubated, but on re-examination 4 hours later, he no longer opens his eyes to painful stimuli, his eyes no longer move with doll's maneuver, and he no longer has corneal reflexes. Repeat CT scan shows stable size of ICH but increase in the size of the ventricles and downward mass effect with early uncal herniation.

THOUGHT QUESTIONS

- What are the signs of increased intracranial pressure (ICP)?
- What are the medical and surgical options in this scenario?

The ICP increase in this case is likely because of hemorrhage extension into the ventricles, which causes clotting and disruption of the flow of CSF out of the ventricles into the subarachnoid space. Increased ICP can manifest in several ways, including headache, nausea, vomiting, decreased arousal, and cranial nerve palsies, ultimately leading to coma.

For mild cases of intracranial HTN, medical management is sometimes enough to prevent progression and permanent damage. Osmotic agents such as mannitol and hypertonic saline work by drawing water out of the cerebral tissue, thus decreasing edema and ICP. Acutely, lowering the PCO_2 by hyperventilation can decrease ICP by stimulating cerebral vasoconstriction. Pentobarbital coma can lower ICP by decreasing cerebral metabolism and thus cerebral blood flow. In the case above, it would be appropriate to initiate one of these therapies even before a CT scan is performed as increased ICP with herniation is the most urgent possible complication. These are all temporizing measures, however, and cannot maintain ICP in the face of ongoing ventricular blockage. An external ventricular drainage (EVD) device or ventriculostomy can be placed at the bedside, which serves both as a direct measure of ICP and as a means of removing CSF (and blood products in this case) to relieve pressure. At present, there is no compelling evidence that more invasive surgical interventions such as hematoma evacuation are helpful in ICH (as opposed to subdural hemorrhage).

CASE CONTINUED

The patient is hyperventilated with some improvement in his exam, and an EVD device is placed emergently. The initial ICP is 24 mm Hg, but after drainage of CSF it lowers to 18. The patient's examination improves slightly.

QUESTIONS

12-1. What is the best predictor of outcome in ICH?
- A. Age
- B. Volume of ICH at presentation
- C. Glasgow Coma Scale (GCS)
- D. Presence of intraventricular hemorrhage

12-2. Which of the following is characteristic of amyloid angiopathy?
- A. Hemorrhages are subcortical.
- B. Patients may show signs of dementia prior to clinically evident ICH.
- C. MRI is not usually helpful in evaluating for this disease.
- D. It is safe for these patients to be on warfarin for other indications.

12-3. What is the initial GCS in the above case?
- A. 12
- B. 8
- C. 4
- D. 0

12-4. What percentage of strokes are primarily hemorrhagic?
- A. 5%
- B. 10%
- C. 50%
- D. 80%

ANSWERS

12-1. B. Volume of hemorrhage at presentation is the best predictor of outcome after ICH. Volume is estimated by the following formula: [volume = (length × width × depth)/2]. Volumes >30 mL have greater mortality and morbidity. Other factors consistently associated with poor outcome are GCS <8, presence of intraventricular hemorrhage, and age >80. Presence of infratentorial hemorrhage has also been associated with worse outcome. Elevated INR at the time of presentation is associated with greater expansion of hemorrhage and with worse outcome, but this effect can be mitigated by prompt reversal of anticoagulation.

12-2. B. Amyloid angiopathy is becoming widely recognized as a cause of ICH in older populations. Amyloid deposition in the cerebral vasculature over time leads to frail blood vessels that rupture more readily. These amyloid deposits are more prevalent in patients with signs of dementia, and patients with Alzheimer's disease have a greater risk of ICH from amyloid angiopathy than other patients, although not all patients with amyloid angiopathy have dementia. MRI susceptibility sequence is sensitive for blood products, including hemosiderin deposits, which may give evidence of prior microhemorrhages. These hemorrhages are more common in the cortex, as opposed to the deep hemorrhages in chronic HTN. Because the blood vessels are more friable and prone to rupture, anticoagulation is generally contraindicated in these patients. If unavoidable, use of warfarin should be closely monitored so as not to reach supratherapeutic levels.

12-3. B. The GCS is a standardized scale of neurologic status, which is useful for documenting a patient's status in emergency settings. The scale is based on three categories as follows in Table 12-1.

In this case, the patient opens eyes to pain (2 points), produces unintelligible sounds (2 points), and withdraws to painful stimuli (4 points), for a GCS = 8. The lowest possible score is 3, and the maximum is 15. While there are more details in the full coma examination, the GCS offers a quick assessment of overall status, and as noted above, can help predict outcome.

TABLE 12-1   Glasgow Coma Scale

	Eye Opening	Verbal	Motor
6	—	—	Obeys
5	—	Oriented	Localizes to pain
4	Spontaneous	Confused	Withdraws to pain
3	To speech	Inappropriate	Flexion (decorticate)
2	To pain	Unintelligible	Extensor (decerebrate)
1	None	None	None

12-4. B. ICH makes up 10% of all strokes, with a prevalence of 37,000 cases per year in the United States, or 12 to 15 cases per 100,000. It is twice as prevalent as subarachnoid hemorrhage. The incidence increases exponentially with age, with rates doubling every 10 years after the age of 35 years.

ADDITIONAL SUGGESTED READING

Greenberg SM. Cerebral amyloid angiopathy: prospects for clinical diagnosis and treatment. Neurology 1998;51:690–694.

Manno EM, JLD Atkinson, JR Fulgham, et al. Emerging Medical and Surgical Management Strategies in the Evaluation and Treatment of Intracerebral Hemorrhage. Mayo Clin Proc 2005;80:420–433.

Headache

ID/CC: 22-year-old female with headaches.

HPI: CM is a 22-year-old right-handed female with a history of headache (HA). Her HA began 9 months ago. Initially they would occur sporadically, every few months, but in the past 1 to 2 months they have been more frequent, occurring once a week. Nausea is a common symptom with her HA, and frequently, she has had a few episodes of emesis. The HA itself consists of throbbing pain over her temple, always on one side. OTC analgesics provide some relief. What helps the most is "sleeping the headache off" in a dark and quiet room. She describes no other neurologic symptoms.

PMHx: Seasonal allergies

Meds: Claritin

All: Penicillin

FHx: History of HA in mother and maternal aunt

SHx: Youngest of five siblings. About to enter medical school.

PE: Gen: Anxious appearing, but otherwise appears well. CV/lungs/abdomen: normal on examination.

VS: WNL

Neuro: Entirely normal

THOUGHT QUESTION

- How will you evaluate the patient's HA?

HAs are a common complaint that bring patients in to seek medical attention. The essential step in evaluating HA is to be able to differentiate between a benign HA and a HA because of an underlying, potentially serious disease process.

In the evaluation of a patient with HA, history should include details such as: frequency, duration of HA, evolution over time (individual HA as well as pattern of HA in general), location of pain, associated symptoms, nausea, other Neurologic or non-neurologic symptoms (weakness, loss of vision, ataxia), relieving or aggravating factors, and detailed family and other medical history.

Some of the factors that suggest benign HA are chronic HA that do not change much over time, identifiable triggers for HA, and family history of HA. It is the chronic or subacute and progressive HAs that are of concern for underlying (potentially) serious CNS pathology (see questions below).

Another way to classify HA has been described in children/ adolescents by Rothner, based on their temporal pattern as:

- Acute generalized (systemic infection, toxic-metabolic causes, cerebrovascular accidents)
- Acute localized (dental infections, sinusitis)
- Acute recurrent (migraine, cluster)
- Chronic progressive (intracranial space occupying lesion, hydrocephalus)
- Chronic nonprogressive (tension HA, postconcussion, depression)

This patient's history suggests benign type of HA. Using Rothner's classification, this is most likely an acute recurrent pattern of HA.

CASE CONTINUED

The patient also reports that during the HA she cannot tolerate loud sounds or bright lights. Often prior to the onset of her HA she sees bright lights in front of her eyes, at times as if light is zigzagging across her fields of vision.

A diagnosis of migraine with auras (classic migraine) is made.

THOUGHT QUESTION

■ What are the principles of treatment?

The principles of treating migraine are:

1. Avoidance of triggers for the HA
2. Acute treatment of an individual attack
3. Prevention of recurrent attacks

Acute treatment of an individual attack (abortive treatment) is accomplished by using analgesics (acetaminophen, aspirin, non-steroidal anti-inflammatory drugs), sumatriptan and related drugs, ergot preparations, or at times a short course of steroids. Opiates should be avoided, but may be used in severe pain. Treatment of accompanying nausea with appropriate antiemetics and hydration (IV if necessary) are adjunctive measures in acute treatment.

Preventive treatment consists of medication taken on a daily basis, with the goal to reduce frequency of HA over time or ameliorate them completely. Examples of drugs used for preventive treatment include β-blockers, tricyclic compounds such as amitriptyline, calcium channel blockers, certain anti-epileptic drugs, methysergide, and cyproheptadine (favored in children).

QUESTIONS

13-1. Which one of the following symptoms or circumstances is less likely to indicate the presence of a more serious underlying etiology of the HA?
   A. Headaches that awaken the patient at night
   B. Failure of OTC drugs to provide relief from HA
   C. Headache worse with sneezing
   D. New-onset HA in a 55-year-old woman
   E. Hiccups

13-2. Common "triggers" for migraine are:
A. Ripened cheeses
B. Red wine
C. Chinese food
D. Chocolate
E. All of the above

13-3. Which drug is commonly used as a preventive treatment for migraine?
A. Valproate sodium
B. Phenobarbital
C. Phenytoin
D. Carbamazepine
E. Trileptal

13-4. A 47-year-old male with intense HA, lacrimation, and congestion in one eye is likely to have the following type of HA:
A. Common migraine
B. Classic migraine
C. Cluster HA
D. Subarachnoid hemorrhage
E. Trigeminal neuralgia

 ANSWERS

13-1. B. In the evaluation of HA, the following factors should raise concern about a serious etiology underlying the HA:
New-onset HA in middle-age or elderly patients
Progressively worsening HA
HAs that wake up a patient from sleep
HA made worse by Valsalva maneuvers
Abnormal neurologic examination
Associated illnesses and systemic signs such as weight loss, anorexia

13-2. E. Foods are associated with migraine. Foods such as ripened cheese, red wine, Chinese food (containing monosodium glutamate), and chocolate are known associations. Not everyone with migraine can identify a specific food trigger. But food sensitivity with regards to HA should form part of the history, as avoiding those foods can help ameliorate HA.

13-3. A. The four drugs mentioned in the choices are all primarily used in the treatment of epilepsy. Valproate sodium is used as a prophylactic or preventive treatment of migraine.

13-4. C. The clinical picture described here is cluster HA. It is seen more commonly in males. Severe pain, which is commonly retro-orbital, may be accompanied by ipsilateral nasal congestion, lacrimation, conjunctival injection, and rarely an ipsilateral Horner's syndrome. Such HAs last under an hour, and as the name implies occur one to three times a day during a cluster. A cluster may last for a few months, followed by a period of remission of months to years.

 ADDITIONAL SUGGESTED READING

Lipton RB, Bigal ME, Steiner TJ, et al. Classification of primary headaches. Neurology 2004;63:427.
Silberstein SD. Practice parameter: evidence-based guidelines for migraine headache (an evidence-based review): report of the quality standards subcommittee of the American Academy of Neurology. Neurology 2000;55:754.

Headache and Vomiting

ID/CC: 15-year-old female with headaches

HPI: PC, a 15-year-old left-handed female presents with headaches. They began 2 weeks prior to her evaluation. Her headaches ware described as throbbing, involving the entire head. They occur daily and are worst in the morning upon waking up. As the day progresses, the headaches get a little better. Acetaminophen and ibuprofen provide some relief. In addition she also has had nausea, vomiting, and intermittent diplopia for 2 days.

PMHx: Acne, asthma

Meds: Minocycline

All: Sulfonamides

FHx: An aunt died of a brain tumor in her 50s

SHx: Straight A student, oldest of four siblings

VS: Afebrile, BP 110/70 HR 80

Exam: HEENT: facial acne. Neck: supple, no meningismus. CV/ lungs/abdomen: normal.

Neuro: Mental status: alert, uncomfortable from pain

**Cranial
nerves:** Pupils reactive

Fundi: Bilateral papilledema. Right sixth nerve palsy. Remainder of cranial nerve examination: normal.

**Motor
examination:** Normal strength

Reflexes: Normal, plantar response flexor bilaterally. Normal coordination and gait.

THOUGHT QUESTIONS

- What is the differential diagnosis?
- What test(s) would you perform?

This patient presents with acute onset headaches. Key features of her presentation are headaches worse upon awakening, nausea, and diplopia. The finding of papilledema on examination is indicative of increased intracranial pressure. This finding in the setting of acute headaches raises the concern of an intracranial space-occupying lesion. Other conditions to be considered are chronic headache disorders like migraine, and pseudotumor cerebri.

In the above setting, the acute onset of headache and papilledema is concerning. A quick screening test to look for a space occupying lesion is a head CT. An MRI scan is better at assessing the presence of tumors, particularly posterior fossa lesions, but is difficult to obtain at short notice.

CASE CONTINUED

A contrast-enhanced MRI scan of the brain is obtained, and is normal. A LP is performed and 30 mL CSF is drained. The opening pressure is 54 cm of H_2O. CSF protein is 10 mg/dL, glucose 46 mg/dL, RBC 0, WBC 1. Gram stain and culture are negative. Closing pressure at the end of the LP is 32 cm of H_2O.

After the LP, the patient's headache improves considerably. Her N&V resolve over the next 1 to 2 days; diplopia gets better and resolves over the next week.

THOUGHT QUESTION

- How do these tests and findings help in the diagnosis?

The normal MRI scan excludes a space-occupying intracranial lesion from the differential diagnosis. The acute presentation, papilledema, and sixth nerve palsy are all signs of raised intracranial pressure. The pattern of headaches is not typical of migraines.

Elevated intracranial pressure is confirmed on the LP. CSF analysis is normal, thereby making an infectious or inflammatory process unlikely.

The presence of papilledema, normal neuroimaging (lack of a space-occupying lesion), and elevated CSF opening pressure constitute the condition of pseudotumor cerebri (benign intracranial HTN).

QUESTIONS

14-1. Which of the following conditions are not associated with pseudotumor cerebri (PTC)?
   A. Hypothyroidism
   B. Hypervitaminosis A or D
   C. Steroid use
   D. Pregnancy
   E. All of the above

14-2. Normal opening pressure of CSF is less than:
   A. 5 cm H_2O
   B. 10 cm H_2O
   C. 15 cm H_2O
   D. 20 cm H_2O
   E. 25 cm H_2O

14-3. Medications used in treating PTC include:
   A. Aspirin
   B. Acetazolamide
   C. Clopidogrel
   D. Dilantin
   E. Propanolol

14-4. Complications of PTC include:
   A. Visual field defects
   B. Herniation
   C. Spinal headache
   D. Meningitis
   E. Long-term cranial neve palsies

ANSWERS

14-1. C. PTC is seen in several systemic conditions, although the most common cause remains idiopathic PTC. Common etiologies include: endocrine abnormalities such as hypo- or hyperthyroidism, cortisol abnormalities, hypervitaminosis A and D, pregnancy, obesity, and systemic diseases like systemic lupus erythematosus (SLE). Medications associated with this condition are tetracyclines (chronic use as in acne), steroids (used chronically), and fat-soluble vitamins. Diabetes mellitus itself is not associated with PTC.

14-2. D. Normal opening pressure of CSF is less than 20 cm of water. It should be measured in the lateral decubitus position, with the patient relaxed, and legs extended.

14-3. C. Diuretics such as furosemide and acetazolamide are used to treat PTC. They are believed to work by decreasing CSF production (acetazolamide is a carbonic anhydrase inhibitor). Although implicated as an etiologic factor, steroids have also been used to treat PTC. Sometimes a single LP provides symptomatic relief, at other times serial LPs are needed. In medically refractory cases, surgical treatment with a lumboperitoneal shunt may be indicated. Optic nerve fenestration has also been described as a procedure to treat PTC.

14-4. A. Visual field defects may be permanent sequelae from untreated PTC. Follow-up of PTC requires monitoring of the patient's peripheral vision by formal visual field testing.

ADDITIONAL SUGGESTED READING

The Brain Trauma Foundation. The American Association of Neurologic Surgeons. The Joint Section on Neurotrauma and Critical Care. Critical pathway for the treatment of established intracranial HTN. J Neurotrauma 2000;17:537.

Lane PL, Skoretz TG, Doig G, et al. Intracranial pressure monitoring and outcomes after traumatic brain injury. Can J Surg 2000;43:442.

Blurry Vision and Headache

ID/CC: 80-year-old man with right frontal headache

HPI: TA is an 80-year-old right-handed male referred for evaluation of headache and blurry vision in the right eye. Patient was doing well until about 4 weeks ago when he started to have right frontal headaches. He has had never had any previous history of headaches. He had no nausea, vomiting, stiff neck, fevers, or photophobia. However, he has felt increasingly fatigued. He has also had blurry vision in his right eye without any double vision or loss of vision. When asked, he reports that his mouth becomes tired when he is eating a meal.

PMHx: HTN, hyperlipidemia, and coronary artery disease

PSHx: Negative

Meds: Aspirin, atenolol, simvastatin

All: NKDA

FHx: Noncontributory

SHx: Retired plumber. No history of smoking or alcohol use

PE: Gen: VS normal. Ophthalmologic examination completely normal including visual acuity and slit lamp examination.

Neuro: Mental status: normal orientation and attention

CN II–XII: Intact. Extraocular movements are full, pupils are equal and reactive without any afferent pupillary defect, visual fields are full, normal funduscopic examination.

Motor exam: Tone: normal. Strength 5/5 in right upper and lower extremities, 5/5 in left upper and lower extremities.

Reflexes: Normal

Cerebellum: No dysmetria or ataxia

THOUGHT QUESTIONS

- What is the differential for this headache?
- What, if any, laboratory tests should I order?
- Does this patient need any neuroimaging?

When evaluating a patient with headache, it is first important to determine if the presentation is acute, subacute, or chronic. Each of these categories of headache has a differential diagnosis that is different as are the diagnostic and therapeutic pathways. The patient in this case has had a headache for several weeks time. In an elderly person with constitutional symptoms such as fatigue, weight loss, or fevers a systemic process should be considered. New, persistent headaches should also be taken seriously. If any of this historical information is present, neuroimaging is usually indicated, even in the absence of positive examination findings. The differential diagnosis includes mass lesion such as malignancy, chronic blood, indolent infection, or another inflammatory process. This patient also complains of blurry vision. It is important to differentiate between blurry vision, double vision, and loss of vision. Patients may often report that their symptoms are present in one eye or another, but it is important to ask whether or not they covered either eye and to examine each eye with the other covered.

Temporal arteritis can be a serious cause of headaches in the elderly, especially in the setting of constitutional and visual symptoms. Patients may complain of jaw claudication, or fatigue while chewing. Patients may also complain of shoulder and arm pain, but not weakness, if the inflammatory response has started to affect the arteries closer to the aortic arch. The temporal artery should be closely examined for tenderness, and the single most important lab measurement is the erythrocyte sedimentation rate.

CASE CONTINUED

Lab: CBC: WNL, electrolytes, glucose, LFTs: WNL. ESR: 70 mm. T4 and TSH: WNL

Imaging studies: MRI brain: Chronic, nonspecific white matter changes. No mass lesion, infarct, or blood.

QUESTIONS

15-1. What is the treatment for temporal arteritis?
A. Prednisone
B. IV immunoglobulin (IVIG)
C. Plasmapheresis
D. Watchful waiting
E. Doxycycline

15-2. How is the final diagnosis of temporal arteritis made?
A. Magnetic resonance angiography
B. LP
C. ESR
D. Ultrasound
E. Biopsy

15-3. The temporal artery is a branch of which parent artery?
A. External carotid artery
B. Internal carotid artery
C. Ophthalmic artery
D. Subclavian artery
E. Maxillary

15-4. What vasculitis should be considered if the patient was a 35-year-old female from Japan?
A. Temporal arteritis
B. Takayasu arteritis
C. Primary central nervous system vasculitis
D. Wegener's disease
E. Churg-Strauss's disease

ANSWERS

15-1. A. Steroids are the primary mode of therapy for patients with temporal, or giant cell, arteritis. They have broad ranging effects on immune responses from T and B cells. Treatment with steroids can be followed clinically and with the ESR. It is needed to avoid potential complications such as vision loss or stroke.

15-2. E. If the clinical suspicion is high, temporal arteritis can be treated without a biopsy. However, in cases of an unclear diagnosis, and an equivocal ESR, a biopsy is often needed. Depending on the surgeon, bilateral biopsies can be performed as well.

15-3. A. The superficial temporal artery is one of the terminal branches of the external carotid artery. The other branches, as they come off the ascending external carotid artery, are superior thyroid, ascending pharyngeal, lingual, facial, occipital and posterior auricular. The maxillary artery is the other terminal branch.

15-4. B. Takayasu arteritis typically presents in women younger than the age of 40 years. There is an increased prevalence in individuals of Asian descent. While granulomatous changes are often present, as in temporal arteritis, the affected vessels are more commonly the aorta and its branches instead of the external carotid artery and its branches. Wegner and Churg-Strauss vasculitis often involve the pulmonary and renal systems.

ADDITIONAL SUGGESTED READING

Salvarani C, Cantini F, Boiardi L, et al. Medical progress: polymyalgia rheumatica and giant cell arteritis. N Engl J Med 2002;347:261–271.

Weyand CM, Goronzy JJ. Mechanisms of disease: medium and large vessel vasculitis. N Engl J Med 2003;349:160–169.

Headache and Progressive Right-Sided Weakness

ID/CC: 28-year-old man with headache and right face and arm weakness

HPI: RA is a homeless man with a history of untreated HIV diagnosed 4 years earlier. He presents to urgent care clinic with a complaint of headache and right arm weakness for the past 2 weeks. The headache is diffuse and dull. The weakness has become gradually worse, such that for the past 2 days he has been unable to write with his right arm. The last time he presented to clinic 2 months prior, his CD4 count was 125 cells/μL and his viral load was 65,000. He is not on antiretroviral treatment (ART) as a result of poor compliance. He has a prescription for trimethoprim-sulfamethoxazole (TMP-SMX) for PCP prophylaxis, but reports he does not take it regularly. He denies any fevers, back pain, or seizures.

PMHx: HIV, h/o oral thrush

PSHx: 0

Meds: TMP-SMX

All: NKDA

FHx: Adopted

SHx: Homeless, unemployed

Habits: No tobacco, occasional alcohol, IVDU with cocaine

VS: Temp 99.1°F BP 110/70 HR 78 RR 12

PE: Disheveled, cachectic, no rash; supple neck, no lymphadenopathy; clear breath sounds

Neuro: Left visual field deficit, right facial droop, right arm weakness with increased reflexes on the right

Labs/drug screen: Screening labs reveal normal basic chemistries, slightly elevated AST and ALT, normal hematocrit, low WBC at 3, and normal platelet count.

THOUGHT QUESTIONS

- What is the differential for CNS mass lesions in HIV patients?
- What diagnostic studies could help narrow the differential?

The differential diagnosis for CNS mass lesions in patients with HIV depends on the level of immunocompromise. In patients with CD4 counts >500 cells/μL, CNS lesions are the same as in normal immunocompetent patients. With CD4 counts between 200 and 500 cells/μL, HIV patients may exhibit some neurologic manifestations, but CNS mass lesions are uncommon. When CD4 counts reach below 200 cells/μL, the most common CNS mass lesions are toxoplasmosis, primary CNS lymphoma, and progressive multifocal leukoencephalopathy(PML). Less common causes include brain abscesses with staphylococcus or other bacteria, syphilis, and—in the developing world—neurocysticercosis and tuberculosis. While sryptococcus more often causes a meningitis in HIV patients, it can sometimes cause a granulomatous mass lesion.

The first step in diagnosis is to obtain neuroimaging. Both CT and MRI are useful, and studies should be done both with and without contrast to determine if the lesion enhances. CT can be obtained quickly and with lower cost to determine if the lesion is exerting dangerous mass effect. However, MRI is more sensitive to smaller lesions, which can be important in determining whether the lesions are multifocal or solitary, and it is better for imaging the posterior fossa.

CASE CONTINUED

CT with and without contrast revealed multiple ring-enhancing lesions, the largest in the left basal ganglia and occipital regions (Figs. 16-1 and 16-2). It also showed surrounding edema indicating mass effect, but no midline shift or herniation. CD4 count comes back at 100 cells/μL.

THOUGHT QUESTIONS

- What is the most likely diagnosis based on imaging characteristics?
- What ancillary studies could you perform to help confirm the diagnosis?

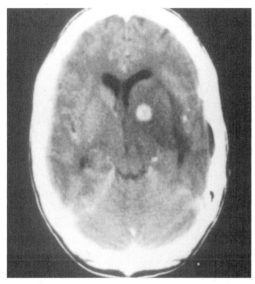

FIGURE **16-1**
Contrast-enhanced CT scan with typical ring-enhancing lesions of cerebral toxoplasmosis. (*From Harwood-Nuss A, Wolfson AB, et al. The Clinical Practice of Emergency Medicine, 3rd Ed. Philadelphia: Lippincott, Williams & Wilkins, 2001.*)

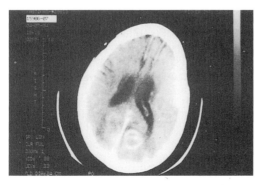

FIGURE **16-2**
Computed tomographic scan of the brain of a patient with toxoplasmic encephalitis shows a ring-enhancing lesion. (*From Sun T. Parasitic Disorders: Pathology, Diagnosis, and Management, 2nd Ed. Baltimore: Lippincott, Williams & Wilkins, 1999.*)

While there are no pathognomonic radiographic findings, the above findings are most consistent with toxoplasmosis. Lesions are typically multifocal, affecting the frontal and parietal lobes, as well as the deep gray matter. Lesions usually enhance in a ring pattern, and surrounding edema is the norm. The other common cause of CNS lesion with mass effect is primary CNS lymphoma. These lesions can be either multifocal or solitary and usually display irregular or patchy enhancement, although ring-enhancement can sometimes be seen. PML typically causes bilateral multifocal demyelination of the subcortical and periventricular white matter, and appears hypodense on CT and T1-weighted MRI, or hyperdense on T2-weighted MRI. Lesions of PML do not typically enhance or cause mass effect.

Serologic testing for antitoxoplasma immunoglobulin G (IgG) antibody can be helpful but is not in itself diagnostic as many patients are exposed to toxoplasma without developing CNS toxoplasmosis. CSF protein, glucose, and cell counts are nonspecific. However, PCR for Epstein-Barr virus (EBV) (associated with CNS lymphoma in the HIV population) and JC virus (causative agent in PML) can be useful in confirming those diagnoses in the right radiographic setting. The standard diagnostic confirmation in patients with suspected toxoplasmosis without impending problems from mass effect is to empirically treat for toxoplasma and repeat imaging in 2 weeks to determine if the lesions have improved.

CASE CONTINUED

The patient is admitted to the hospital and initiated on a regimen of sulfadiazine and pyrimethamine, with folinic acid to counter the bone marrow toxicity of pyrimethamine. The patient is also counseled on the importance of ART, but it is not started at this time. After 2 weeks, repeat MRI shows improvement in the size and enhancement of the lesions. The patient is continued on the same regimen at lower doses for long-term suppression.

QUESTIONS

16-1. If there were no response to empiric toxoplasma treatment, what would be a reasonable next step?

A. Initiate steroid treatment
B. Repeat LP
C. Perform brain biopsy
D. None of the above

16-2. Which of the following symptoms are also seen with CNS toxoplasmosis?

A. Seizures
B. Fever
C. Confusion
D. All of the above

16-3. CNS complications of cytomegalovirus (CMV) include which of the following?

A. Retinitis
B. Ventriculo-encephalitis
C. Micronodular encephalitis
D. All of the above

16-4. The most useful diagnostic study to confirm cryptococcal meningitis in the acute setting is:

A. MRI with and without gadolinium
B. CSF fungal cultures
C. CSF cryptococcal antigen
D. CSF India ink smear

ANSWERS

16-1. C. Brain biopsy is the definitive test for CNS mass lesions. The procedure carries risk of morbidity, and can be avoided if there is improvement with empiric toxoplasmosis treatment. If there is no improvement, biopsy is necessary to direct specific treatment. Steroids should be avoided until after biopsy, as they can reduce the yield from biopsy. There is no utility in repeating an LP in this case.

16-2. D. CNS toxoplasmosis causes symptoms based on its size, location, edema, and mass effect. As it can affect the cortex, seizures are a common manifestation, as are focal motor and sensory disturbances. It can also cause nonspecific symptoms such as fever and confusion.

16-3. D. CMV affects the CNS by reactivation when CD4 counts drop below 50 cells/μL. Early complications include retinitis, esophagitis, or colitis. CMV can cause confusion and focal abnormalities by a ventriculo-encephalitis with inflammation and enlargement of the ventricles apparent on neuroimaging, or through a diffusely scattered micronodular encephalitis. The prognosis is extremely poor for either form, with death occurring usually within weeks to months.

16-4. C. Cryptococcus most commonly causes a meningitis in HIV patients with CD4 counts <200 cells/μL. MRI may show leptomeningeal enhancement, but this is nonspecific. Fungal cultures of CSF are the gold standard, but may take weeks to come back. India ink smear is helpful if positive, but is insensitive. CSF cryptococcal antigen is a rapid test and is more than 90% sensitive. If positive, treatment options include amphotericin B with or without flucytosine.

 ## ADDITIONAL SUGGESTED READING

Koralnik IJ. Approach to HIV-infected patients with central nervous system lesions. UpToDate, www.uptodate.com; access June 2006.

Verma A. Neurologic manifestations of human immunodeficiency virus infection in adults. In: Bradley WG, et al, eds. Neuro Clin Pract 2004;59:1581–1602.

Headache and Lethargy

ID/CC: 54-year-old man with a history of lung cancer who presents with complaint of headache and lethargy for 2 months.

HPI: MC was diagnosed with lung cancer 1 year ago. At that time, he underwent resection of the lesion and adjuvant chemotherapy with a negative metastatic work-up. Two months ago, the patient developed headaches described as "a dull overall ache occurring daily." These symptoms are occasionally associated with N&V. Two days ago he developed significant weakness in his left leg. The family also reports that over the last few weeks he has become more lethargic and is easily fatigued. He remains intact cognitively and is able to perform all his activities of daily living.

PMHx: Lung cancer

PSHx: Thoracotomy for resection of left lung lesion

All: NKDA

Meds: None

SHx: Tobacco—100 pack per year history. He quit 1 year ago. No alcohol, no IVDA or illicit drug use.

FHx: The patient's father died of a brain tumor.

VS: BP 142/68 HR 77 RR 12

PE/Neuro: The patient is awake and in no acute distress. His cranial nerves are intact. He has significant weakness in all the motor groups of the left lower extremity—3/5 plantar and dorsiflexion, 4/5 medial and lateral hamstrings. His ankle reflexes are 3 bilaterally and there is an extensor plantar response on the left (Babinski reflex).

Contrast head MRI: Solid, 1.5-cm, well-circumscribed contrast-enhancing lesion in the right frontal lobe. There is associated peritumoral edema (Fig. 17-1).

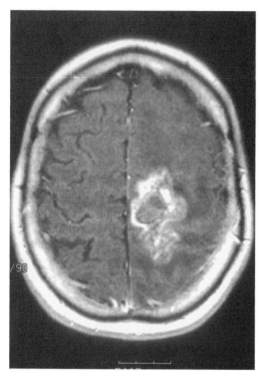

FIGURE 17-1
Contrast head MRI:
Solid, 1.5-cm well-
circumscribed
contrast-enhancing
lesion in the right
frontal lobe. There
is associated peritu-
moral edema.
(*Image provided by
the Departments of
Neuroradiology
and Neurosurgery,
Stanford University,
Stanford, California.*)

THOUGHT QUESTIONS

■ What is the patient's differential diagnosis?
■ How would you proceed at this time?

The history, PE, and radiographs are consistent with either a primary CNS brain tumor or a metastatic lesion from the patient's lung primary. With a history of lung cancer, a diagnosis of cerebral metastasis is more likely.

The next step in the evaluation of this patient is to repeat the metastatic work-up including a CT scan of the chest and abdomen. The presence of additional metastatic lesions may alter treatment options and choice of adjuvant therapy.

CASE CONTINUED

The metastatic evaluation does not reveal any additional lesions. The patient is placed on anticonvulsants and corticosteroid taper. Treatment options are discussed with the family and a craniotomy with resection of the lesion is performed. The patient tolerated the procedure. The pathology demonstrates tumor consistent with a primary of small-cell carcinoma of the lung. The patient is referred to neuro-oncology and radiation oncology. He is scheduled for postoperative radiation therapy.

QUESTIONS

17-1. Which of the following is the most common primary cancer in patients with cerebral metastases?

    A. Renal cell (kidney)
    B. Breast
    C. Lung
    D. Melanoma
    E. Gastrointestinal (GI)

17-2. The increased incidence of cerebral metastases may be a result of which of the following?

    A. Increased ability to diagnose CNS tumors
    B. Increased survival of cancer patients
    C. Use of chemotherapeutic drugs
    D. Use of radiation
    E. All of the above

17-3. Which of the following types of lung cancer is a common source of metastases?

    A. Small-cell
    B. Mesothelioma
    C. Oat cell
    D. Squamous cell
    E. Other nonsmall cell

17-4. Which of the following is the most common site for metastatic CNS disease?

    A. Cerebral hemispheres
    B. Cerebellum
    C. Brainstem
    D. Thalamus
    E. Basal ganglia

ANSWERS

17-1. C. Metastases are a frequent source of brain tumors, accounting for approximately 50% of all brain tumors. Lung cancer is the most frequent source of brain metastases in adults, accounting for 44% of all cerebral metastases. Other sources of cerebral metastases include renal cell—7%, GI—6%, breast—10%, and melanoma—3%.

17-2. D. Greenberg notes that the relative increase in the incidence of cerebral metastases may be a result of a number of factors including increased length of survival of cancer patients, increased ability to diagnose these tumors because of improvements in imaging modalities (CT and MRI scans), and the use of chemotherapeutic agents that result in an increased ability for CNS seeding by transiently weakening the BBB and agents that are unable to cross the BBB, thus allowing preferential CNS tumor growth.

17-3. A. Small-cell cancer of the lung is the most frequent bronchogenic metastatic cancer. Studies have demonstrated the presence of cerebral metastases in up to 80% of patients with small-cell cancer of the lung. Small-cell cancer of the lung is more radiosensitive than other primary bronchogenic metastatic cancers. As a result, radiation therapy is often administered following surgery.

17-4. A. The majority of all metastases are supratentorial. Approximately 80% of solitary metastases are located in the cerebral hemispheres. The cerebellum is not an uncommon site of intracranial metastases, accounting for 16% of solitary brain metastases. Thus the cerebellum is the most common posterior fossa location of cerebral metastases. Nonetheless, the posterior fossa and brainstem are not the most common sites of such lesions.

ADDITIONAL SUGGESTED READING

Forsyth PA, Weaver S, Fulton D, et al. Prophylactic anticonvulsants in patients with brain tumour. Can J Neurol Sci 2003;30:106.
Wen PY, Loeffler JS. Management of brain metastases. Oncology (Huntingt) 1999;13:941.

IV

Patients Who Present with Altered Mental Status/Memory Loss/Personality Changes

New Onset Dementia

ID/CC: 77-year-old man with 6-week history of difficulty walking, problems with memory, and urinary incontinence

HPI: PD's wife reports that approximately a month and a half ago he developed difficulties with walking. She describes Mr. D as having "great difficulty beginning to walk" and then once he starts, "he shuffles slowly." She also notes that while standing he is unsteady. Approximately 4 weeks ago, Mr. D began to experience urinary incontinence. Since then he has had ever-increasing difficulties with memory and more frequent episodes of incontinence. He was seen first by his primary care physician and has also been evaluated by a neurologist where a complete dementia work-up was performed. A noncontrast head CT demonstrates enlarged lateral ventricles without prominence of cortical sulci. He is referred for continued evaluation.

PMHx: HTN

PSHx: None

Meds: Lasix

All: NKDA

SHx: He is married and lives with his wife and eldest daughter.

VS: Temp 97.9°F BP 142/84 HR 88 RR 16

PE/Neuro: The patient is awake and alert. He is disoriented to date. He has difficulty with both recent and immediate recall on memory testing. Remote memory is intact. The patient scores 23 out of 30 on the MMSE.

His neurologic exam demonstrates spasticity and hyperreflexia in the upper and lower extremities. He has bilateral grasp reflexes. The plantar responses are extensor bilaterally. He has no weakness in either his upper or lower extremities. He has marked difficulty initiating gait. His gait is slow and shuffling.

Labs: WNL

**Noncontrast
head CT:**   Enlarged lateral ventricles without prominence of cortical sulci (little atrophy) (Fig. 18-1).

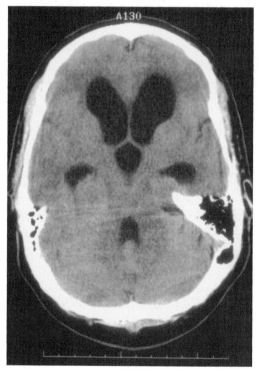

FIGURE 18-1
Noncontrast head CT: Enlarged lateral ventricles without prominence of cortical sulci (little atrophy).
(*Image provided by the Departments of Neuroradiology and Neurosurgery, Stanford University, Stanford, California.*)

THOUGHT QUESTIONS

- What is the patient's differential diagnosis?
- What diagnostic test would you order at this time?

     The differential diagnosis includes conditions producing dementia. These include normal-pressure hydrocephalus, Alzheimer's disease, Parkinson's disease, and multi-infarct dementia. The history and radiographic images are most consistent with normal-pressure hydrocephalus. (See answer to questions below for details.)

Alzheimer patients usually have a longer period of symptoms (months to years versus weeks to months). Additionally, the CT and MRI of patients with Alzheimer's disease usually demonstrate enlarged cortical sulci. Patients with Parkinson's disease may have similar radiographs, but these patients usually have profound extrapyramidal signs of rigidity and tremor. Patients with multi-infarct dementia usually have a history of cerebrovascular disease and strokes, and usually present with focal neurological signs.

A LP would be appropriate at this time. (See answer section below for details.)

CASE CONTINUED

A LP is performed in the clinic. The opening pressure (OP) is 175 mm H_2O. The CSF protein, glucose, and cell count are WNL (see chart below). Approximately 50 mL of CSF is removed. At the next clinic visit the patient's wife reports that following the procedure, she noticed a transient improvement in gait and memory and a decrease in incontinent episodes. Treatment options are reviewed with the family and the decision is made to place a VP shunt.

QUESTIONS

18-1. Which of the following is the classic triad of normal pressure hydrocephalus?
- A. Dementia, focal weakness, and urinary incontinence
- B. Aphasia, ataxia, and urinary incontinence
- C. Dementia, ataxia, and urinary incontinence
- D. Neglect, aphasia, and urinary incontinence
- E. Dementia, ataxia, and dysmetria

18-2. Which of the following is usually the initial manifestation of normal pressure hydrocephalus?
- A. Dementia
- B. Gait apraxia
- C. Presence of pyramidal signs
- D. Retropulsion
- E. Urinary incontinence

18-3. Which of the following LP opening pressures, as the upper limit, is consistent with nephronophthisis (NPH)?
A. 100 mm H_2O
B. 150 mm H_2O
C. 200 mm H_2O
D. 300 mm H_2O
E. 350 mm H_2O

18-4. Which of the following radiographic studies or clinical tests is pathognomonic for NPH?
A. Enlarged ventricles on CT scan
B. Absence of cerebral atrophy on CT scan
C. Improvement in gait following LP
D. Improvement after CSF shunt is placed
E. None of the above

ANSWERS

18-1. C. Dementia, gait apraxia, and urinary incontinence are all part of the classic triad of normal-pressure hydrocephalus. The presence of pyramidal signs is a frequent finding on neurologic examination, but is not part of the triad.

18-2. B. Gait disturbances are usually the first manifestation of normal-pressure hydrocephalus.

18-3. B. The normal opening pressure is <180 mm H_2O. A normal or low OP with LP is consistent with NPH.

18-4. D. There is no clinical test or radiographic imaging that is pathognomonic for normal-pressure hydrocephalus. The history, PE findings, radiographic imaging, and response to removal of CSF on LP must all be considered. The best predictor of a favorable clinical response to shunting is transient improvement in gait and memory and decrease in incontinent episodes after removal of 30 to 50 mL of CSF during a LP.

In this patient the decision was made to place a VP shunt. In all cases this decision should be made only after a thorough neurologic evaluation and dementia work-up. There are no guarantees for improvement. The best responders are those presenting with the classic triad of symptoms, an opening pressure on LP that is between 100 mm H_2O to 180 mm H_2O and CT or MRI with communicating hydrocephalus but without cortical atrophy. Those patients shunted after a shorter period of time also have a better chance of improvement postshunting.

VP shunts have several non-negligible complications. These include infections, subdural hematomas, and shunt malfunctions. They may be experienced by as many as one-third of the patients (Table 18-1).

TABLE **18-1**   CSF Composition (Normal Values)

Opening pressure	60 mm H_2O–180 mm H_2O
Protein	10–45 mg/dL
Glucose	40–80 mg/dL
Total leukocyte	<5/mm^3
Cell count	0–5 lymphs/HPF

 ADDITIONAL SUGGESTED READING

Caselli RJ. Current issues in the diagnosis and management of dementia. Semin Neurol 2003;23:231.
Cummings JL. Alzheimer's disease. N Engl J Med 2004;351:56.
Press DZ. Parkinson's disease dementia—a first step? Engl J Med 2004;351:2547.

Memory Loss and Personality Changes

ID/CC: 68-year-old man is brought in by his wife and son for increasing mood swings and forgetfulness.

HPI: JD's problems began several years ago. He owns a heating and air conditioning business where he had worked together with his two sons. Several years ago he began having angry outbursts at work, which was very uncharacteristic for him. Over the last year they have become more frequent and one son, with whom he is no longer on speaking terms, has left to start his own business. The other son reports the fights usually begin when his father forgets what he has told his employees and thinks that things that have been done still need to be done. The patient says that he is somewhat embarrassed by the angry outbursts but insists that his son is wrong, that he has not forgotten anything, and that his anger is justified. His wife reports similar problems at home. He has not physically harmed anyone but his wife has become afraid of him during his outbursts. Once a reputable, bright, and kind businessman, his son tells you in private, the patient is no longer performing well at work because of his forgetfulness and anger and the business is suffering.

PMHx: HTN, CAD

PSHx: Coronary stent placement and angioplasty 4 years ago

Med: Atenolol, simvastatin and ASA 81 mg four times a day

All: NKDA

SHx: Heavy smoker since age 19, quit 6 years ago. World War II veteran. Lives with his wife. Does not drink alcohol.

FHx: HTN and heart disease; most family members died before age 70 years. No history of neurodegenerative disorders or strokes.

Neuro Hx: No history of head injury, blackouts, or seizures. No slowness of movement, abnormal movements, or tremors.

THOUGHT QUESTIONS

- How would you summarize the case thus far?
- What is the differential diagnosis?
- What are the most likely diagnoses and what risk factors does he have for each?

This is a previously intellectually normal elderly man who presents with chronic, progressive onset of personality changes and memory loss. An important feature to note for management purposes is his potential for violence. Personality changes (and other neuropsychiatric symptoms) are often the first symptom of a neurodegenerative illness and may precede the onset of memory loss and/or movement abnormalities by months to years. His clinical features are consistent with a dementing illness.

The differential diagnosis for a chronic, progressive dementing illness includes primary degenerative dementias (Alzheimer's disease [AD], Pick's disease, frontal lobe dementia, and frontotemporal dementia), vascular dementias (multi-infarct dementia, dementia following a single stroke, subcortical arteriosclerotic encephalopathy), dementia because of infections (HIV, spirochetal disease, chronic viral encephalitides), metabolic disorders (hypothyroidism, vitamin B12 deficiency, dialysis dementia, hepatocerebral degeneration), neoplasms (midline tumors such as colloid cysts, pinealomas, pituitary tumors, or midline gliomas), drugs and toxins (alcohol, arsenic, and mercury), repeated head trauma (also known as dementia pugilistica), multiple sclerosis, normal pressure hydrocephalus, and pseudodementia because of severe depression. Additionally, dementia is a common feature of several degenerative movement disorders such as Parkinson's disease, diffuse Lewy body disease, supranuclear palsy, Huntington's disease, and corticobasal degeneration. These are usually easily distinguished on PE by the presence of movement abnormalities.

The most likely case, given his age and risk factors and the prevalence of these diseases are AD and multi-infarct dementia (MID). His age and sex are a risk factor for both and his history of coronary atherosclerotic disease and smoking are risk factors for MID.

CASE CONTINUED

VS: Temp 98.6°F BP 130/70 HR 76 RR 16

PE: Gen: Unremarkable. No carotid bruits. No lymphadenopathy. Lungs: CTA. COR: RRR no murmurs. Abdomen: soft, nontender, nondistended, no organomegaly.

Neuro: MSE: Patient is well-groomed and cooperative. His mood is "okay" and affect appears appropriate. No psychomotor slowing or agitation is present. MMSE 22/30 with impaired memory, language, and constructional ability and intact attention testing.

CN II–XII: Intact.

Motor: Normal strength and bulk throughout. Moderately increased tone in all four extremities with no asymmetry.

Reflexes: 2+ throughout. Babinski signs absent bilaterally. Rooting reflex is present. Absent grasping and palmomental reflexes.

Sensory: Intact to light touch, pinprick, temperature, and vibration throughout.

Coordination: No tremor, dysmetria, or nystagmus is present.

Gait: Normal, no ataxia, and intact tandem gait.

Labs: CBC, LFTs, electrolytes, BUN, creatinine, vitamin B12, thyroid function tests, and heavy metal screen all WNL

Imaging studies: Brain MRI shows global cerebral atrophy and small, periventricular, T2 hyperintense abnormalities. No gadolinium enhancement or corresponding T1 lesions are seen.

QUESTIONS

19-1. What type of language deficit is the patient likely to develop?
   A. Aphasia resembling a Wernicke aphasia
   B. Aphasia resembling a Broca aphasia
   C. Asphasia resembling a transcortical sensory deficit
   D. Aphasia resembling a transcortical motor deficit
   E. Orofacial dyspraxia with speech production deficits

19-2. What are the pathologic hallmarks of this disease?
A. Degeneration of the nucleus basalis
B. Neurofibrillary tangles
C. Cerebrovascular amyloid
D. Senile plaques
E. All of the above

19-3. What additional work-up should be done?
A. Apolipoprotein E genotyping
B. Carotid Dopplers
C. LP
D. PET scan of the brain
E. Neuropsychological testing

19-4. How should this patient be managed?
A. Mood-stabilizing drug (lithium, carbamazepine, or valproate)
B. Antidepressant
C. Acetylcholinesterase inhibitors
D. A and C
E. All of the above

 ANSWERS

19-1. C. Language disturbances (dysphasia) and visuospatial problems in addition to memory impairment are the clinical hallmarks of AD. PE findings are often normal but extrapyramidal abnormalities are frequently observed as in this patient. Primitive reflexes (grasp, rooting, and sucking) can also be found but do not correlate with the degree of cognitive impairment. The language disturbance will resemble a transcortical sensory aphasia as the disease progresses. Transcortical sensory aphasia is a fluent aphasia with good repetition and poor comprehension. In AD patients the aphasia differs slightly in that some degree of impaired verbal fluency is usually present and that confrontational naming, particularly of semantic groups, is also impaired (e.g., "name as many animals as you can think of in the next minute"). Orofacial dyspraxia with speech production deficits and eventually echolalia and palilalia are characteristically involved in advanced frontal lobe–dominant Pick's disease.

19-2. D. Brain atrophy with neuronal loss and neurofibrillary tangles predominating in the CA1 layer of the hippocampus, subiculum, layers 2 and 5 of the entorhinal cortex, and layers 3 and

5 in the neocortex are characteristic findings in AD although not exclusive to this disease. Neurofibrillary tangles are composed at least in part of paired helical filaments. Senile plaques are made up of a central core of β-amyloid surrounded by dystrophic neuritis and glial processes and are found predominantly in association areas of the cerebral cortex. The observation that dropout of cholinergic neurons and neurofibrillary tangles occurs also in the nucleus basalis of Meynert (the source of most of the cholinergic projections to the cerebral cortex) led to a major breakthrough in the symptomatic management of AD. Other pathologic characteristics of AD include cerebrovascular amyloid, Hirano bodies, and granulovacuolar degeneration of neurons.

19-3. E. No further work-up is needed. The work-up in AD is directed at excluding potentially reversible causes of dementia. While the presence of the E4 allele of apolipoprotein E has been linked to some familial AD cases and appears to contribute to age of onset and amyloid load in sporadic AD (earlier onset, higher amyloid load), it has been shown to be only a risk factor for AD, not causative. Therefore, screening him or his family members for the E4 allele will not provide any useful information, especially because there are currently no protective treatments available. While PET or single-photon emission computed tomography (SPECT) scans would likely show bilateral temporoparietal hypometabolism and hypoperfusion, they are ordered only when there is a high degree of suspicion that this is another type of primary neurodegenerative dementia and should be ordered by a dementia expert.

19-4. D. Management of AD is directed at symptomatic relief and control. Management of the neuropsychiatric symptoms of AD (depression, delusions and hallucinations, personality change, and behavioral disturbances) comprises the major component of medical treatment of AD patients. This patient shows behavioral disturbance (aggression) and needs to be treated and monitored carefully. Should he become physically aggressive he should be placed in a supervised facility immediately for his wife's protection. Treatment of verbally aggressive behavior as in this patient usually begins with a mood-stabilizing agent but may require the addition of an anxiolytic and antipsychotic depending on the progression and cause of the outbursts. While 25% to 30% of AD patients require treatment of depression, this patient does not currently exhibit any symptoms. The use of anticholinesterase inhibitors (tacrine and donepezil) has been shown to improve global and memory function early in the course of AD as in this patient. Tacrine can cause significant elevation of liver transaminases and therefore liver function tests must be monitored regularly.

ADDITIONAL SUGGESTED READING

Boustani M, Peterson B, Hanson L, et al. Screening for dementia in primary care: a summary of the evidence for the U.S. Preventive services task force. Ann Intern Med 2003;138:927.

Petersen RC, Stevens JC, Ganguli M, et al. Practice parameter: early detection of dementia: mild cognitive impairment (an evidence-based review). Report of the Quality Standards Subcommittee of the American Academy of Neurology. Neurology 2001;56:1133.

Teri L, Logsdon RG, Peskind E, et al. Treatment of agitation in AD: a randomized, placebo-controlled clinical trial. Neurology 2000; 55:1271.

Headache and Personality Changes

ID/CC: 46-year-old HIV-positive man is brought in by his partner for evaluation of fatigue, headache, and change in personality.

HPI: Several months ago, AD began complaining of increasing fatigue, followed shortly thereafter by headache. His partner also reports that Mr. D has become increasingly "depressed" and no longer wants to see their friends or leave their apartment. Last week his partner came home to find him confused and disoriented. This resolved over several hours. On several occasions he has also had difficulty remembering to take his medications, which his partner now has to arrange for him. On neurologic review of systems, the patient complains of a slight tremor and imbalance, which he says is the reason he no longer wants to go out. He denies feeling dysphoric, but does complain of anorexia and insomnia that began several months ago. He has lost 10 pounds over the last 3 months. His last CD4 count was <200 cells/μL 3 months ago.

PMHx: HIV for 15 years. No acquired immune deficiency syndrome (AIDS)–defining illnesses. Chronic pedal fungal infection.

PSHx: Arthroscopic knee surgery at the age of 35 years.

Meds: Antiretroviral regimen

All: NKDA

SHx: Homosexual, no history of IVDA, lives with his longtime partner who is also HIV. Receives regular care in a specialized HIV clinic and is compliant with medications. He was employed full-time until 1 month ago as an accountant but has taken a medical leave of absence.

FHx: No history of stroke, dementia, tremor, or seizures

Neuro Hx: Toxic peripheral neuropathy from prior retroviral therapy diagnosed by EMG/NCV and nerve biopsy. No history of seizures or head injuries.

THOUGHT QUESTIONS

- How would you summarize the case thus far?
- What is the differential diagnosis?

The case can be summarized as a middle-aged HIV-positive man with a history of drug-induced polyneuropathy with a subacute onset of memory loss, depression, headaches, mild tremor, and imbalance and more recently episodes of confusion. Memory loss is a common finding in dementing illnesses and encephalopathies. Depression is a common comorbid condition in patients suffering from dementing illnesses and encephalopathies. However, primary major depression with impaired concentration can mimic dementia, often known as pseudodementia. The headaches could be a result of the dementing process/encephalopathy or unrelated, the mild tremor and imbalance could be a result of focal neurologic lesions or part of the degenerative process, and the episodes of confusion could represent seizures, transient global amnesia, TIAs, or acute worsening of the encephalopathy.

The differential diagnosis for subacute onset of an encephalopathy/dementing illness in an HIV-positive or HIV-negative patient includes: (1) infectious causes such as a chronic encephalitis (usually viral) or chronic meningitis (granulomatous disease, tuberculosis, fungal), both of which could also account for the headaches; (2) vascular disease such as multiple infarcts (often from embolic sources associated with endocarditis), primary or secondary CNS vasculitis; (3) endocrinologic and nutritional deficiencies (hypothyroidism, vitamin B12 deficiency, Wernicke encephalopathy); (4) prion disease (this has a rapidly progressive course); (5) psychiatric or drug-induced depression (primary depression or depression secondary to medications such as β-blockers, or drug-induced encephalopathy as can sometimes be seen with the use of antiepileptics); (6) tumor or trauma (chronic subdural hematomas often present in this manner); and (7) primary neurodegenerative illnesses such as Alzheimer's disease, Pick's disease, Huntington's disease, and corticobasal degeneration, although the onset of these illnesses is usually slower.

Other diagnoses that occur most commonly in HIV-positive and AIDS patients and could account for his symptoms include: toxoplasmosis, primary CNS lymphoma, progressive multifocal leukoencephalopathy, HIV-associated dementia, CMV encephalitis, cryptococcal meningitis, and neurosyphilis.

 CASE CONTINUED

VS: Temp 98.6°F BP 110/70 HR 68 RR 16

PE: Gen: Patient is disheveled and poorly groomed. He appears slender but not cachectic. No lymphadenopathy, alopecia, or skin lesions are noted. Lungs are clear to auscultation. COR: RRR no murmurs. Abdomen is soft and nontender with no organomegaly.

Neuro: MSE: His affect is flat, mood is "okay." Significant psychomotor slowing is present. Speech is clear and coherent but slowed and monotonous. He is unable to do serial sevens, but can recite the days of the week backwards, albeit with a significant amount of delay. He is disoriented to date only. The remainder of his MMSE is intact.

CN II–XII: Intact.

Motor: General slowing of motor movements. Fine motor skills are slowed and moderately imprecise but asymmetry is noted. Strength and bulk are normal in all four extremities. Tone is slightly decreased in the lower extremities.

Reflexes: 1 in the upper extremities and at the patella. Absent in the ankles. Babinski signs present bilaterally.

Sensory: Diminished light touch, pinprick, and vibration in a symmetrical stocking distribution. The remainder of his sensory examination is intact.

Coordination: Diminished facial expression. Abnormal saccadic eye movements and lack of smooth pursuit. No nystagmus is present. A fine, regular, postural tremor is noted in both upper extremities. No dysmetria is present.

Gait: Slightly wide based and ataxic

Lab: Brain MRI with and without gadolinium shows large, T2 hyperintense, nonenhancing lesions in the centrum semiovale and the right parietal lobe without mass effect. CSF results are as follows: increased immunoglobulin G (IgG); WBC, 15 cells/µL;

98% mononuclear cells; 2% PMNs; RBC 5 cells/μL; protein, 80 mg/dL; and glucose, 48 mg/dL. Peripheral blood CD4 count is 150 cells/μL.

QUESTIONS

20-1. What work-up should be ordered next?
A. Brain biopsy
B. CSF PCR for Jakob-Creutzfeldt (JC) virus
C. Syphilis serology
D. EEG
E. All of the above

20-2. Suppose a brain biopsy is ordered. What would you expect it to show?
A. Multinucleated giant cells and astrocytosis
B. Neurofibrillary plaques and tangles
C. Demyelination, giant astrocytes, and oligodendrocytic inclusion bodies
D. Lewy bodies
E. Perivascular inflammatory infiltrates with intracytoplasmic neuronal inclusion bodies

20-3. What would be an appropriate treatment in addition to his current antiretroviral treatment?
A. Zidovudine (AZT) 1000 mg by mouth four times a day
B. Stavudine 40 mg by mouth twice a day
C. Antidepressant
D. Ativan
E. All of the above

20-4. Suppose the MRI showed generalized cerebral atrophy, sulcal widening, and ventricular dilatation with no other abnormalities present. What would the most likely diagnosis be?
A. HIV-associated dementia
B. Early Alzheimer's disease
C. Meningovascular syphilis
D. Diffuse lymphoma
E. Progressive multifocal leukoencephalopathy

ANSWERS

20-1. E. The patient's signs and symptoms are highly sugges-tive of a global dementing illness associated with some mild motor and coordination impairments. None of the PE findings suggest a focal deficit other than his old peripheral neuropathy (gait abnor-mality, diminished reflexes and stocking distribution loss of sensa-tion). The combination of bradyphrenia, bradykinesia, and clumsiness is strongly suggestive of HIV-associated dementia or PML. PML can also present with focal deficits in addition to these findings. The characteristic finding on CT or MRI scan for PML is a nonenhancing, demyelinating lesion without mass effect in the centrum semiovale, parieto-occipital lobes or cerebellum. PML is caused by reactivation of JC virus and can sometimes be diagnosed by evidence of JC virus in the CSF by PCR. However, the definitive diagnosis can be made by only brain biopsy of the lesion. An EEG should be ordered to determine whether this patient should be treated for seizures, given the history of episodes of confusion. In all HIV patients presenting with nervous system disease, syphilis serology should be sent as neurosyphilis can mimic a number of the HIV-related neurologic illnesses and can be more readily treated.

20-2. C. Demyelination, giant astrocytes, and oligodendrocytic inclusion bodies are the hallmarks of PML. The tissue is also usually stained for JC virus using immunostaining, electron microscopy, or in situ hybridization. Multinucleated giant cells and astrocytosis are the characteristic findings in HIV-associated dementia, and neurofibrillary plaques and tangles are seen most often in Alzheimer's disease. Perivascular inflammatory infiltrates with intracytoplasmic neuronal inclusion bodies are usually seen with viral infections such as CMV encephalitis. CMV encephalitis almost never occurs in patients with CD4 counts greater than 100 cells/μL.

20-3. C. Approximately 5% of all AIDS patients will develop PML and in 25% of these patients PML is the AIDS-defining illness. The prognosis is extremely poor, with only a 5% to 10% 1-year survival and most patients dying within 4 months of diagnosis. Currently, treat-ment with intrathecal or IV cytosine arabinoside (AraC) has been tried with mixed results. High-dose AZT and, if this fails, stavudine are the appropriate treatments for HIV-associated dementia. This patient does suffer from somatic complaints attributable to depression and should be treated appropriately. Depression with the absence of dysphoria in PML and HIV-associated dementia is common.

20-4. A. The characteristic MRI findings of HIV-associated dementia (also called HIV subacute encephalitis, HIV encephalopathy, and AIDS dementia complex) early in the disease are just generalized atrophy reflected by the sulci widening and ventricular dilatations. As the disease progresses, multifocal patchy or punctate subcortical white matter lesions become apparent, which may later become confluent. These lesions usually occur in the periventricular regions, particularly at the frontal and occipital horns. HIV-associated dementia is the most common neurologic complication of AIDS. It occurs in 15% to 20% of AIDS patients and may be the AIDS-defining illness. In addition to apathy, psychomotor retardation, and memory loss, the patients often develop impaired fine motor coordination, frontal release signs, tremor, and myoclonus. Extensor plantar reflexes (Babinski sign) are a common finding and seizures can also occur.

Other neurologic complications associated with HIV infection can be broken down into two main categories: (1) those that are a direct result of HIV infection, and (2) those that are indirectly related to HIV. Directly related to HIV infection are vacuolar myelopathy, peripheral neuropathy (usually sensory but can also be demyelinating or autonomic), inflammatory myopathy, and cranial neuropathies (Bell's palsy). Indirectly related to HIV infection are opportunistic infections, cranial metastases from lymphoma or Kaposi's sarcoma, vascular disease such as hemorrhages caused by thrombocytopenia or vasculitis as a result of herpes zoster, and peripheral neuropathies or mitochondrial myopathy because of antiretroviral therapies.

 ADDITIONAL SUGGESTED READING

Davis HF, Skolasky RL Jr, Selnes OA, et al. Assessing HIV-associated dementia: modified HIV dementia scale versus the Grooved Pegboard. AIDS Read 2002;12:29.

Dunlop O, Bjorklund R, Bruun JN, et al. Early psychomotor slowing predicts the development of HIV dementia and autopsy-verified HIV encephalitis. Acta Neurol Scand 2002;105:270.

Developmental Regression in Childhood

ID/CC: 18-month-old child presenting with loss of milestones

HPI: ML is an 18-month-old child seen for developmental concerns. He had just started a new day-care program, and the teachers there thought that he was falling more than usual for his age and level of activity. He seemed quiet, but the teachers couldn't tell if it simply was because he was adjusting to his new environment. Over several weeks it becomes more apparent, even to his parents, who had not seemed to notice it initially. When the falling first started, he had an 18-month well-child check by his pediatrician, and was given a clean bill of health. Over the next several weeks, his parents agreed that he was not learning new words as quickly, and that he seemed less interested in his books and toys.

Birth Hx: He was born following an uncomplicated pregnancy and labor. Birth weight and neonatal course were normal. He met his early developmental milestones on time, and his development had seemed normal until he began appearing delayed a few months ago.

PMHx: Healthy child, few URIs and otitis media while in day-care

Meds: None

All: None

FHx: Noncontributory

SHx: Parents first cousins. Two normal, older sisters.

VS: WNL. Weight 12 kg. Head circumference 48 cm.

PE: Gen: unremarkable

Neuro: Alert, makes eye contact. Cranial nerves: intact.

Motor: Decreased muscle tone, particularly in lower extremities. Deep tendon reflexes diminished. Able to walk, but gait unsteady.

THOUGHT QUESTIONS

- What is your differential diagnosis? (broad categories)
- How does the examination aid in the differential diagnosis?

Developmental delay is a common cause for referral to a pediatric neurologist. While assessing developmental delay in a child, it is of utmost importance to determine whether there is simply delay in attaining milestones in some or all areas of development, or whether previously acquired milestones have been lost. Work-up and differential diagnosis are directed accordingly. Degenerative disorders with regression of development have different patterns of presentation. The most common and obvious presentation is a child with apparently normal development who then slows down or plateaus in development and over time begins losing ground. Regression may be apparent in cognitive or motor skills depending upon the disease. In severe diseases that present at birth, or have presumed prenatal onset, there may be no obvious development and the infant may appear to have a static encephalopathy. Some degenerative diseases present in adolescence or adulthood, in which case the motor or cognitive regression is obvious from the start.

At first glance, this child may appear to be one in whom developmental delay has been noticed at 18 months. However, the history is clear that this child achieved normal milestones up to a point and then his development reached a plateau and began regressing. Given such a history one must consider a degenerative process affecting the central nervous system high on the differential diagnosis. That the child's parents are cousins raises the possibility of an autosomal recessive disease.

The examination helps to determine what type of degenerative disorder one might be dealing with (see questions below). Findings on general examination may also provide clues to the nature of the disease. Table 21-1 lists some examples.

TABLE **21-1** Clues to Degenerative Diseases on General Examination

General Examination	Degenerative Disease	General Examination	Degenerative Disease
Macrocephaly	Alexander's disease Canavan's disease Tay-Sachs's disease	Cutaneous abnormality (e.g., hypo/ hyperpigmented macules)	Tuberous sclerosis Neurofibromatosis Ataxia-telangiectasia
Microcephaly	AIDS Rett's syndrome	Skeletal abnormalities	Mucopoly-saccharidosis
Hepatomegaly	Tay-Sachs's disease		Multiple sulfatase deficiency
Splenomegaly	Mucopolysaccharidosis Peroxisomal disorders Glycogen storage diseases	Deafness (especially early in the disease)	Peroxisomal disorders Mitochondrial disorders Certain organic acidemias
Retinal cherry red spot	Tay-Sachs's disease Niemann-Pick's disease	Kinky hair	Refsum disease Menke disease
Other ocular abnormalities	Wilson's disease (Kayser-Fleischer ring) Mucopolysaccharidosis (corneal clouding) Homocystinuria (lens dislocation) Cataracts (galactosemia)		

CASE CONTINUED

Imaging: MRI scan: Abnormal white matter signal, mild cerebral atrophy (Fig. 21-1)

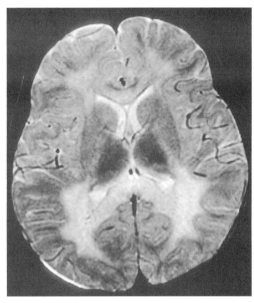

FIGURE 21-1
MRI scan (axial T2 image) of the brain, showing extensive periventricular white matter abnormality. (*Image courtesy of Dr. D.M. Olson, Stanford University Medical Center, Stanford, California.*)

Labs: Basic chemistries: WNL. Given the white matter abnormalities, a number of metabolic studies were sent. Leukocyte enzyme studies reveal a deficiency in Aryl sulfatase A.

A diagnosis of metachromatic leukodystrophy was made.

Individual neurodegenerative disorders are rare conditions, but taken as a whole they are not that uncommon in a pediatric neurologist's practice. It is important to be aware of these disorders, as they are (mostly) inherited conditions and arriving at a specific diagnosis can have a tremendous impact on a family.

QUESTIONS

21-1. Features of a predominantly white matter disease are:
   A. Seizures
   B. Ataxia
   C. Spasticity
   D. Myoclonus
   E. Cognitive decline

21-2. Features of a predominantly gray matter disease are:
A. Deafness
B. Optical atrophy
C. Myoclonus
D. Spasticity
E. Cortical blindness

21-3. Work-up of a possible degenerative disorder in a child must include:
A. Neuroimaging studies
B. Ophthalmologic evaluation
C. Metabolic studies
D. Family history
E. All of the above

21-4. Which of the following is a degenerative disease?
A. Autism
B. Tay-Sachs's disease
C. Sickle cell disease
D. Kawasaki's disease
E. Duchenne's disease

 ANSWERS

21-1. C, **21-2.** C. Early in the course, a given degenerative disease may affect the gray or white matter first. This can be an important clue in steering the work-up. Clues to white matter disorders are: deafness, visual decline (optic atrophy/cortical blindness), spasticity, hyperreflexia, and Babinski sign. Peripheral neuropathy may be present in some. Clues to gray matter disorders are: seizures, ataxia, myoclonus, and cognitive decline. These distinctions become less obvious as a disease progresses, and eventually there is gray and white matter involvement in most diseases.

21-3. E. Neuroimaging studies are important in identifying white matter abnormalities, atrophy, and other specific structural abnormalities. MRI scan (with spectroscopy where available) is the neuroimaging study of choice. Ophthalmologic examination is also important, especially to identify certain storage diseases. Look for optic atrophy or peculiar findings in the retina.

Metabolic studies help identify specific diseases as enzyme assays are available for diagnosing several metabolic diseases. Screening metabolic tests can help identify what type of disease the clinician is dealing with and tailor the work-up.

21-4. B. Tay-Sachs's disease, the mucopolysaccharidosis, and Batten's disease are all examples of degenerative conditions. Autism is a disorder of language and social skills.

 ADDITIONAL SUGGESTED READING

Glascoe FP. Early detection of developmental and behavioral problems. Pediatr Rev 2000;21:272.

Shevell M, Ashwal S, Donley D, et al. Practice parameter: evaluation of the child with global developmental delay: report of the Quality Standards Subcommittee of the American Academy of Neurology and The Practice Committee of the Child Neurology Society. Neurology 2003;60:367.

CASE **22**

Episode of Confusion

 ID/CC: 84-year-old right-handed man is brought in by his daughter following an episode of confusion.

HPI: MS was on the phone with his daughter when he suddenly began speaking gibberish. The daughter repeatedly tried to ask him questions but his responses were inappropriate. After 10 minutes he began speaking normally again. Initially the patient denied the episode but now states that he remembers hearing his daughter and trying to answer her questions but the words would not come out right. He denies any headache, fatigue, nausea, or weakness during or after this episode. He has not started any new medications within the last 2 months.

PMHx: CAD, HTN, osteoarthritis

PSHx: Four-vessel CABG 5 years prior

Meds: Atenolol 50 mg twice a day, Tylenol with codeine as needed, niacin, ASA 81 mg four times a day

All: NKDA

SHx: He is widowed and lives alone. He would prefer to live with his daughter. His daughter would like him to enter an assisted living facility, which he refuses and is what they were arguing about when the episode occurred.

FHx: Heart disease

Neuro Hx: None

THOUGHT QUESTIONS

■ What is your differential diagnosis? (at least three possibilities)

118

■ What signs will you look for on examination to aid in diagnosis?

■ Name the major functional subdivisions of the frontal lobe and clinical symptoms associated with lesions in these areas.

The differential diagnosis for an acute, brief episode of altered mentation in the elderly should include seizure, TIA, transient global amnesia, medication side effect, undiagnosed dementia, and psychological precipitants.

On examination important signs to look for are abnormalities in language testing including a sample of writing, detailed MMSE, subtle weakness on the right side, carotid bruits, cardiac murmur, and evidence of microthrombi or increased intracranial pressure on funduscopic exam.

The frontal lobe includes the (1) primary somatomotor cortex, (2) premotor cortex, (3) motor speech cortex, and (4) prefrontal cortex (often subdivided into the anterior and orbital areas).

The primary somatomotor cortex receives most of its input from the premotor area, somatosensory cortex, and posterior ventrolateral thalamus. Its output makes up 40% of the heavily myelinated, fast-conducting fibers of the pyramidal tract. Isolated lesions of the primary somatomotor cortex (precentral gyrus) result in a flaccid contralateral paralysis; however, most diseases affecting this area also affect the adjacent premotor area, resulting in a spastic paralysis.

The premotor cortex has afferent and efferent connections to the anterolateral ventral thalamus through which it is connected with the basal ganglia and cerebellum. It is essentially the cortical representation of the extrapyramidal system. This area controls the synergistic contraction of functionally related muscle groups and relaxation of antagonistic muscles to be able to carry out complex motor movements; coordinates the involuntary movement of head and trunk with eye movements; and controls voluntary eye movements and "reflex" complex motor movements such as hitting the brakes when a deer jumps out in front of you. Destructive lesions in this area can cause a variety of deficits ranging from the loss of such involuntary motor "reflexes," disequilibrium with frequent falls (connection with the cerebellum), and conjugate gaze deviation toward the side of the lesion. Irritative lesions (focal epilepsy) cause conjugate gaze, head, and neck deviation away from the side of the lesion.

Damage to the motor speech area in the dominant hemisphere results in a cortical motor aphasia where the patient is able to understand words and has normal vocal strength, but is unable to coordinate the motor movements necessary to produce speech (he is mute).

Damage to the prefrontal cortex, or frontal association areas, produces two distinct clinical syndromes resulting from damage to either the anterior frontal lobe or orbital frontal lobe.

Anterior frontal lobe damage results in a decline in initiating motor activity and slowness of mentation. The patients become socially withdrawn and family members often complain that they "just sit there" doing nothing. It is often confused with depression and catatonia but the patients usually are unaware of these problems. Common causes are strokes, tumors, trauma, and neurodegenerative diseases. Orbital frontal lobe damage is characterized by a loss of social inhibitions despite intact intellectual functioning. The patients usually have no insight into their condition. Although they have difficulty holding onto jobs and may encounter problems with the law because of minor offenses (public urination, exposure, etc.), they are not violent.

   CASE CONTINUED

VS: Temp 98.6°F BP 120/70 HR 76 RR 16

PE: Gen: No carotid bruits or cardiac murmur are auscultated.

Neuro: MMSE: 29/30—missed recall of one object after 5 minutes. Speech is fluent, coherent, and appropriate, as is a sample of his written language.

CN II–XII: Intact. Funduscopic examination is normal. Visual fields are full. EOMI, PERRLA, facial strength, and sensation are symmetrical, palate and uvula elevate symmetrically; gag reflex is intact; sternocleidomastoid strength is equal bilaterally.

Motor: Strength, bulk, and tone are normal in all four extremities. Rapid alternating movements and fine motor coordination are symmetrical in both hands. Muscle stretch reflexes are equal and symmetrical, two at triceps, biceps, brachioradialis, and patella and one at Achilles. Babinski signs are absent bilaterally.

Sensory: Intact to light touch and pinprick throughout, slightly diminished vibration sensation in toes bilaterally, intact at the ankles.

Coordination: No tremor, dysmetria, or dysdiadochokinesis is observed.

Gait: Ambulates with a walker because of severe osteoarthritis in his knees. No ataxia is present.

 QUESTIONS

22-1. Based on his history and PE what is the most likely diagnosis?
- A. Seizure
- B. Transient ischemic attack
- C. Transient encephalopathy
- D. Dementia
- E. Psychological etiology

22-2. What should your work-up include?
- A. Cardiac ECHO
- B. Carotid Dopplers
- C. Lipid panel
- D. CT scan of the brain
- E. All of the above

22-3. What is his risk of having a disabling stroke in the next 5 years?
- A. 5%
- B. 10%
- C. 30%
- D. 50%
- E. 70%

22-4. His carotid Doppler shows an 80% narrowing of the left carotid artery and a 60% narrowing on the right. His cardiac ECHO shows no evidence of intracardiac thrombi. Assuming his cardiologist clears him for surgery, what should you recommend?
- A. Left carotid endarterectomy
- B. Bilateral carotid endarterectomies
- C. No intervention
- D. Anticoagulation therapy only
- E. Antiplatelet therapy only

ANSWERS

22-1. B. TIA typically occur in the elderly and last less than 20 minutes, after which recovery is full without any postictal symptoms as in this patient. He did not have any alteration in consciousness, making a seizure or encephalopathy extremely unlikely. The description of the event is typical of a Wernicke aphasia. His MMSE is normal, thus dementia is also extremely unlikely. While psychological causes such as anxiety or an attempt to manipulate his daughter are common in the elderly, this is a diagnosis of exclusion. The briefness of this episode and his initial denial also argue against this. Another important factor is his history of CAD, a risk factor for cerebral atherosclerotic disease.

22-2. E. The work-up for a TIA should include carotid Dopplers to rule out significant stenosis, a cardiac ECHO to rule out an intracardiac thrombus, and at minimum a CT scan to look for evidence of previous ischemic disease. An EEG is not necessary. Other tests should include a CBC and ESR to rule out a giant cell arteritis.

22-3. C. Up to one third of patients with a TIA will have a disabling stroke within the next 5 years. Most of these will occur within the first year following a TIA, the highest period of risk being within the first few weeks following the TIA. Therefore, prompt work-up and treatment are imperative in patients with TIAs.

22-4. A. The risk of stroke from an asymptomatic carotid stenosis of 60% or greater is 11% over 5 years and surgery should be reserved for those who are expected to live longer. For symptomatic carotid stenosis of 70% or greater, carotid endarterectomies have been shown to be superior to medical management except in the case of a complete occlusion, in which case the surgery must be performed within 24 hours of occlusion or the results may be detrimental. He should clearly undergo surgery for the symptomatic stenosis (left) and be placed on antiplatelet therapy following the surgery. Because of the high risk of morbidity and mortality associated with carotid endarterectomies, surgery should be performed only at specialized centers with intraoperative EEG monitoring capabilities by a surgeon with a low complication rate.

ADDITIONAL SUGGESTED READING

Elie M, Rousseau F, Cole M, et al. Prevalence and detection of delirium in elderly emergency department patients. CMAJ 2000;163:977.

McCusker J, Cole M, Dendukuri N, et al. The course of delirium in older medical inpatients: a prospective study. J Gen Intern Med 2003;18:696.

Confusion in an Elderly Man

ID/CC: 58-year-old man presents with confusion.

HPI: AJ was found in a confused state, stumbling around their apartment by his roommate. His roommate had last seen him 2 days ago, at which time the patient appeared to be in his normal state of health. The patient is inattentive but alert and is able to follow a few simple commands. He does not appear to recognize his roommate and is completely disoriented.

PMHx: Several episodes of pneumonia over the last 7 years

PSHx: None

Meds: None

All: NKDA

SHx: He has been unemployed for more than 10 years. Divorced with two children. Has consumed one fifth of hard liquor a day for more than 20 years. Smokes 1 PPD for 40 years. No history of illicit drug use.

FHx: Unknown, he has no contact with any of his siblings or children.

Neuro Hx: History of alcohol withdrawal seizures and blackouts in the past

THOUGHT QUESTIONS

- What is your differential diagnosis?
- What are some neurologic complications of alcoholism? (at least five possibilities)

■ What laboratory tests will you order to aid in your differential diagnosis?

The differential diagnosis at this point still needs to remain broad because the patient cannot provide a history of his symptoms and the roommate was absent for 2 days. The primary complaint is an acute encephalopathy, which can be a result of: (1) metabolic derangements, such as hypoglycemia, uremia, hyper- and hypocalcemia, hepatic encephalopathy, hyponatremia, and thiamine deficiency; (2) CNS infection (encephalitis or meningitis); (3) trauma (subdural hematomas are common in alcoholics); (4) systemic infections, particularly pulmonary infections, which can lead to hypoxia, and in the case of fungal lung infections are often associated with intracerebral lesions; (5) toxicities such as alcohol poisoning, carbon monoxide, illicit drugs, and heavy metals; (6) vascular disease such as intracerebral or subarachnoid hemorrhage and bilateral infarctions; and (7) hypoxic encephalopathies because of severe cardiac failure (alcoholism can cause a dilated cardiomyopathy, pneumonia, or COPD exacerbation).

Neurologic complications of chronic alcoholism include alcoholic polyneuropathy, alcoholic dementia, hepatocerebral degeneration (a dementing illness with parkinsonism), cerebellar atrophy, hepatic encephalopathy, alcohol withdrawal seizures, delirium tremens, Wernicke encephalopathy, Korsakoff's syndrome, central pontine myelinolysis, Marchiafava-Bignami's disease, and amblyopia (visual loss caused by a selective optic nerve lesion).

Laboratory evaluation for this patient should include a CBC, electrolytes, BUN creatinine, blood glucose, liver function tests, ABG, urinalysis, ECG, chest radiograph, head CT, serum calcium, phosphate, osmolality, and toxicity screen from urine and blood.

 CASE CONTINUED

VS: Temp 99.6°F BP 140/80 HR 96 RR 16

PE: Gen: Patient's breath smells of alcohol. Lungs are clear to auscultation. COR: RRR with no murmurs. Abdomen is soft, non-tender, and no hepatosplenomegaly is present.

Neuro: MSE: The patient is thin and disheveled. He is alert and able to follow simple verbal commands with repeated requests. He is able to speak and makes brief, inappropriate replies to repeated questions. He is disoriented to person, place, and time. He cannot give accurate personal information such as his social security number, address, or the names of his children.

CN: Blinks to threat in all visual fields, squeezes eyes shut to bright lights. PERRLA, pupils are deviated toward the midline in straightforward gaze. He is unable to abduct either eye on conjugate gaze and when each eye is tested individually, marked horizontal nystagmus on lateral gaze is present. Adduction, upward gaze, and downward gaze are intact. Facial strength and sensation appear equal bilaterally. Corneal and gag reflex are intact. Tongue and uvula are midline.

Motor: He can maintain all limbs against gravity for more than 5 seconds and moves all limbs spontaneously. Tone and bulk appear normal.

Reflexes: 1+ throughout, absent at both ankles, no asymmetry is noted. Babinski signs absent bilaterally.

Sensory: Withdraws all limbs to light stimulus

Coordination: No tremor or asterixis is noted. Patient is unable to cooperate with finger-nose or heel-chin testing.

Gait: Wide based ataxia

Labs: Head CT scan is normal. Chest radiograph and EKG are also normal. The remainder of the labs is pending.

 QUESTIONS

    23-1. How would you describe his eye movement abnormalities?
      A. Bilateral cranial nerve IV palsies
      B. Bilateral cranial nerve palsies
      C. Symmetrical internuclear ophthalmoplegia
      D. Bilateral cranial nerve VI palsies
      E. Bilateral cranial nerve III palsies

23-2. What might you expect a brain MRI to show?
  A. T2 hyper-intensities in the mamillary bodies and in the periventricular zones around the third and fourth ventricles
  B. Confluent T2 hyperintense lesion in the central portion of the corpus callosum
  C. T2 hyperintensity in the central pons
  D. Significant temporal lobe atrophy
  E. T2 hyper-intensities in the periventricular regions around the lateral ventricles and in the pons

23-3. What is the appropriate next step?
  A. Correct hyponatremia no faster than 12 mEq/L per 24 hours
  B. Thiamine 50 to 100 mg IV four times a day, hold all carbohydrates until the first dose is given
  C. 1 amp of dextrose
  D. General IV nutritional supports
  E. IV corticosteroids to reduce edema and inflammation

23-4. Aside from alcoholism, what other conditions can cause this illness?
  A. Refeeding after prolonged fasting or starvation
  B. Anorexia nervosa
  C. Acquired immune deficiency syndrome (AIDS)
  D. Hemodialysis or peritoneal dialysis
  E. All of the above

 ANSWERS

23-1. D. This is a classic description of bilateral sixth cranial nerve palsies (the abducens nerve). At rest the affected eye is medially deviated and with lateral gaze, the affected eye is unable to abduct even when tested individually. Diplopia is particularly severe with sixth nerve lesions because there is no associated ptosis to obliterate the false image. Often the patient will squeeze one eye shut voluntarily and this may mimic ptosis.

23-2. A. The triad of confusion, abnormal eye movements, and ataxia is the hallmark of Wernicke encephalopathy. The acute confusional state usually comes on over days or weeks and the patients are rarely stuporous or comatose. Inattention and memory loss are the hallmarks of their encephalopathy, most likely a reflection of the involvement of the bilateral mamillary bodies.

Although the original description of the eye movement abnormalities in Wernicke encephalopathy was ophthalmoplegia, the most common eye findings are bilateral sixth nerve palsies with horizontal nystagmus on lateral gaze with or without palsies of other extraocular muscles. The diagnosis is based on the clinical triad; there are no definitive laboratory tests available. Although the brain MRI could also be normal, one can sometimes see the areas of acute hemorrhage followed by gliosis in the areas adjacent to the fourth and third ventricle in the medulla, pons, and midbrain as well as lesions or atrophy of the mamillary bodies. A confluent central corpus callosal lesion is the hallmark of Marchiafava-Bignami's disease. Demyelination in the central pons is what might be seen in central pontine myelinolysis. Periventricular lesions around the lateral ventricles and in the pons occur most often in multiple sclerosis.

23-3. B. The appropriate treatment for Wernicke encephalopathy (a consequence of thiamine deficiency) is the administration of IV thiamine prior to the administration of any carbohydrates, dextrose included. If carbohydrate loading precedes thiamine administration it can precipitate an acute worsening of symptoms and often leads to the more permanent condition of Korsakoff psychosis. Slowly correcting a hyponatremia is the correct treatment for central pontine myelinolysis and general nutritional support is the treatment for Marchiafava-Bignami's disease.

23-4. E. Although Wernicke encephalopathy most often affects chronic alcoholics, many cases have occurred in other states that lead to a poor nutritional status including inadequate nutritional supplementation for patients receiving IV feedings because of a variety of primary conditions (hyperemesis gravidarum, esophageal carcinoma, and stomach stapling among others).

Despite treatment with IV thiamine throughout the acute period, the mortality rate of Wernicke encephalopathy remains 10% to 20%.

 ## *ADDITIONAL SUGGESTED READING*

Ely EW, Shintani A, Truman B, et al. Delirium as a predictor of mortality in mechanically ventilated patients in the intensive care unit. JAMA 2004;291:1753.

McCusker J, Cole M, Dendukuri N, et al. The course of delirium in older medical inpatients: a prospective study. J Gen Intern Med 2003;18:696.

Altered Mental Status and Fever

ID/CC: 24-year-old left-handed male presenting with fever, altered mental status.

HPI: BM is a 24-year-old left-handed male brought to the ED for evaluation of altered mental status. Four days prior to presentation, he developed a flulike illness, with fever, myalgia, and headache. He then developed nausea and vomiting. He thought he had the "stomach flu" so stayed at home and tried to drink lots of fluids and rest. However his fever persisted and headache worsened. On the day of presentation, his roommate noticed that he was lethargic, difficult to arouse, and looked more ill than on the days before, so he drove the patient to the ED.

PMHx: Seasonal allergies, recent sinusitis

PSHx: Tonsillectomy as a child

Meds: Claritin

All: None

FHx: Diabetes mellitus in father

SHx: Graduate student, social drinker, occasional marijuana, no IV drug abuse

PE: Gen: Sinus tachycardia, no skin rash, no hepato-splenomegaly

VS: Temp 102°F BP 110/70 HR 120 RR 30

Neuro: Mental status: lethargic. Roused to painful stimulation, pushed examiner's hand away. Followed simple commands such as "stick out your tongue."

Cranial nerve examination: Intact.

Funduscopic
examination: No papilledema

Motor: Moved all extremities to painful stimulation

Reflexes: Symmetric, brisk 3+, with bilateral extensor plantar
responses

Neck: Stiff to passive flexion

THOUGHT QUESTIONS

- What is the differential diagnosis?
- What is a Kernig sign?
- What tests would you order to make a diagnosis?

The patient's condition is an acute encephalopathy. In the setting of a febrile illness, the most likely etiology is an acute infection of the CNS, such as meningitis. A rapidly progressing process like this is most likely bacterial meningitis; but viral meningitis or encephalitis (particularly herpes simplex infections) can present with such a rapid course. Noninfectious, inflammatory conditions such as a vasculitis can present this way as well. Other causes of an acute encephalopathy include:

Subarachnoid hemorrhage: A prodrome of fever, and so on, is less likely. Prominent symptoms would be an intense headache, classically described as the worst headache of the patient's life, photophobia, meningismus, and depending on the source of the bleed, focal neurological signs. A large stroke or space-occupying lesion with cerebral edema could present as altered mental status, again, focal deficits should be obvious on examination, and the time course would be different. Encephalopathies from toxic/metabolic causes are less likely in this situation and the history will help exclude them.

A Kernig sign is a sign of meningeal irritation. To elicit this sign, the patient lies supine. His hip is partially flexed, and then leg extended at the knee. This elicits pain in the back of the leg because of stretching of lumbar nerve roots.

Work-up is directed at establishing the cause of the patient's symptoms and instituting treatment rapidly. Besides the clinical examination, a head CT is required to assess for a bleed, acute stroke, or evidence of raised intracranial pressure that would preclude a LP. A LP is needed, as are basic laboratories like CBC, chemistries, and blood cultures.

CASE CONTINUED

Labs: CBC/WBC: 19,500 with 65% polymorphs, and 10% bands. Chemistries: electrolytes: WNL. Blood glucose 108 mg/dL, renal and liver function tests: WNL

Blood cultures: Pending

Head CT without contrast: Normal

Lumbar puncture: opening pressure: 270 mm H_2O (elevated), protein: 150 mg/dL, glucose: 15 mg/dL, cell count: 2,400 cells, 95% polymorphs. Gram stain and culture: pending.

The patient was put on IV antibiotics and admitted. Supportive treatment (IV fluids, antipyretic measures, etc.) were instituted. Over the next 48 hours, the patient defervesced. His encephalopathy showed progressive improvement.

THOUGHT QUESTION

- How does the CSF picture help to further narrow the diagnosis?

This patient's CSF has an elevated opening pressure, elevated protein, marked reduction in glucose, and pleocytosis with a polymorphonuclear predominance. This picture is most commonly seen in bacterial meningitis. The table below summarizes CSF findings in a few other conditions. Also, the Gram stain is likely to show bacteria in the CSF (Table 24-1).

TABLE 24-1 CSF Findings

	Appearance	Protein (mg/dL)	Glucose (mg/dL)	WBC (/cu mm)	RBC (/cu mm)
Normal (adult)	Clear	15–40	50–70 (1/2–2/3 of blood glucose level)	<5	None-few
Bacterial meningitis	Cloudy or purulent	Elevated (100s)	Low (may be undetectable)	1,000s	Few
Aseptic meningitis	Clear or slight turbidity	10–100	Normal	10s or less	Few
Herpes encephalitis	Cloudy or hemorrhagic	10–100	Normal	100s–1,000s	10–1,000
Subarachnoid hemorrhage*	Hemorrhagic, xanthochromic	100s	Normal or low	100s or less	1,000s (out of proportion to WBCs)

*Normal CSF does not exclude the diagnosis of subarachnoid hemorrhage.

QUESTIONS

24-1. What organism is most likely to grow from the CSF culture?
  A. *Escherichia coli*
  B. Enterovirus
  C. *Listeria monocytogenes*
  D. *Streptococcus pneumoniae*
  E. *Staphylococcus epidermidis*

24-2. Complications from meningitis include:
  A. Abscess formation
  B. Arthritis
  C. Uremia
  D. Sinusitis
  E. Gastritis

24-3. Which of the following organisms is specific for meningitis in the neonatal period?
  A. *Neisseria meningitidis*
  B. *Diplococcus pneumoniae*
  C. Nocardia
  D. Enterobacter
  E. Group B streptococcus

24-4. The spinal interspace entered during a LP is:
  A. L4-L5
  B. L5-S1
  C. L2-L3
  D. S1-S2
  E. L1-L2

ANSWERS

24-1. D. The organism most likely to grow from the patient's CSF culture is *Streptococcus pneumoniae*, a gram-positive diplococcus, which is the most common cause of meningitis in young adults. *E. coli* commonly causes sepsis and meningitis in neonates, *Staphylococcus epidermidis* produces systemic disease in IV drug users (Table 24-2).

TABLE 24-2 Etiology of Bacterial Meningitis by Age Group

Neonates
Group B streptococcus
Escherichia coli
Listeria monocytogenes
Children <15 years
Haemophilus influenzae
Neisseria meningitidis
Streptococcus pneumoniae
Children >15 years and adults
Streptococcus pneumoniae
Neisseria meningitidis
Haemophilus influenzae
Staphylococcus aureus

24-2. A. Meningitis that leads to focal cerebritis can cause abscess formation. Septicemia and pericarditis are systemic complications from meningitis and bacteremia. Chronic sinusitis may be present in patients who develop a frontal brain abscess, but does not occur as a complication of meningitis.

24-3. E. Organisms that cause neonatal sepsis and meningitis are *E. coli*, Group B streptococcus, and *Listeria monocytogenes*. In children and infants *Haemophilus influenzae, S. pneumoniae*, and *S. meningococcus* are common organisms. In adults meningococcus and pneumococcus are more common.

24-4. A. During a LP, the anatomical landmark palpated on the spine is the spinous process of the L4 vertebra. The space above or below is entered for the procedure.

ADDITIONAL SUGGESTED READING

de Gans J, van de Beek D. Dexamethasone in adults with bacterial meningitis. N Engl J Med 2002;347:1549.

Hasbun R, Abrahams J, Jekel J, et al. Computed tomography of the head before LP in adults with suspected meningitis. N Engl J Med 2001;345:1727.

Frontal Sinus Fracture

ID/CC: 32-year-old man who was involved in a motor vehicle accident

HPI: GP was an unrestrained passenger in an automobile that was T-boned on the passenger side. Mr. P was unable to open his eyes, his speech was incomprehensible, he was able to localize painful stimuli. He was intubated for airway protection and brought to the emergency room immidiately via the paramedics.

PMHx: Unavailable

PSHx: Unavailable

Meds: None known

SHx: Unavailable

Habits: None known

VS: WNL

PE: The patient had multiple abrasions of the head and neck. He had bilateral periorbital swelling and ecchymoses. His eyes were swollen shut. There was blood and clear drainage from the nose and a laceration of the lip. He continued to localize briskly to stimuli.

Labs/drug screen: WNL

THOUGHT QUESTIONS

- What is the significance of the PE findings?
- What is the differential diagnosis?

A thorough physical and neurologic examination is extremely important. A high index of suspicion is therefore needed. The presence of peri orbital ecchymosis and drainage from the nose are key clinical findings. Careful examination of the nasoethmoidal region should be carried out to rule out injury. The differential diagnosis includes basal skull fracture and frontal sinus fracture. Both of these diagnoses are associated with significant intracranial injury. The risk is greater with frontal sinus fracture because of the proximity of the frontal sinus to the brain and the great forces required to cause a frontal sinus fracture. A CSF leak should raise the suspicion of disruption of the posterior wall with a dural tear.

CASE CONTINUED

The trauma evaluation included a non-contrast head CT and later dedicated fine cuts of the facial bones and sinuses and a CT of the cervical spine. Both the radiographs and clinical examination of the cervical spine were WNL. There was no evidence of soft tissue injury and there were no fractures noted. The alignment was WNL.

On CT scan of the frontal bones, a complex comminuted fracture of the frontal sinus involving both the anterior and posterior tables of the frontal sinuses. There are also other facial bone and orbital fractures noted. Pneumocephalus is noted throughout the middle and anterior cranial base. There is no intra- or extra-axial blood, no midline shift and no ventricular involvement.

THOUGHT QUESTIONS

- Why was the patient intubated?
- What considerations should be made for the route of intubation?
- In addition to the neurologic examination what other evaluation should be obtained?

As with all trauma patients, standard trauma protocol should be performed with emphasis on ensuring an adequate airway, breathing, circulation, CNS status, and C-spine. The patient was intubated for airway protection. The patient was orally intubated, as a nasotracheal intubation is contraindicated in suspected basal skull fractures.

Thorough neurologic and ophthalmic examination is mandatory in all traumatic injuries of the frontal sinus. Evaluation of visual acuity, pupillary function, ocular mobility and inspection of the anterior chamber for blood and the fundus for disruption are necessary.

   CASE CONTINUED

The patient was brought to the operating room by the neurosurgery and the oral facial maxillary surgery teams. He underwent cranialization and exenteration of the frontal sinus fractures. Additionally, open reduction and internal fixation of the frontal sinus fractures and the facial bone fractures was performed. There were no intraoperative complications.

QUESTIONS

25-1. Which wall of the frontal sinus is the weakest?
   A. Anterior wall
   B. Posterior wall
   C. Equal strength

25-2. What is the most frequent indication for surgical repair of an anterior wall fracture?
   A. CSF leak
   B. Mucocele
   C. Cosmetic deformity
   D. None of the above

25-3. In repairing a displaced posterior wall fracture, which of the following is necessary?
   A. Obliteration of the frontal sinus
   B. Exenteration
   C. Cranialization
   D. All of the above

25-4. Partial or complete obstruction of the nasofrontal duct is associated with which of the following?
   A. Acute and/or chronic sinusitis
   B. Mucocele
   C. Mucopyocele
   D. All of the above

 ANSWERS

25-1. B. The anterior wall is the stronger of the two tables. The posterior wall is much thinner and weaker and separates the sinus from the dura of the frontal lobe in the anterior cranial fossa.

25-2. C. The anterior wall is very rarely associated with CSF leak or injury to the drainage system. Isolated closed fractures involving nondisplaced or minimally displaced anterior wall only do not require operative intervention. All open fractures should be explored to assess the true extent of the injury. Isolated depressed fractures pose a risk for cosmetic deformity. These fractures should be explored for possible reduction and fixation.

25-3. D. Obliteration of the frontal sinus is the recommended treatment for displaced frontal sinus fractures. The rationale is to provide a secure barrier between the unsterile nasal cavity and the intracranial area. Complete removal of the mucosa is imperative to prevent potential mucocele formation. If >50% of the posterior wall is fractured, cranialization is also necessary to provide a vascular bed to support the graft.

25-4. D. A competent nasofrontal communication is necessary to the normal function of the frontal sinus. Partial obstruction of the nasofrontal duct (NFD) may predispose to chronic sinusitis or recurrent episodes of acute sinusitis. Complete obstruction of the NFD can lead to mucocele formation, which may act as an expanding tumor, eroding bone and exerting a mass effect on adjacent brain or orbit. If bacteria seed the mucocele, a mucopyocele will develop with the potential danger of life threatening intracranial infections. Therefore, the surgical treatment of fractures impairing drainage of the frontal sinus requires either reconstruction of the sinus drainage system or obliteration of the sinus.

ADDITIONAL SUGGESTED READING

Swinson BD, Jerjes W, Thompson G. Current practice in the management of frontal sinus fractures. J Laryngol Otol 2004;118:927–932.

Coma

ID/CC: 72-year-old woman presenting with altered mental status.

HPI: CM is a 72-year-old female who presents with altered mental status to the ED, from the nursing home where she is a resident. She was found unresponsive by the nursing staff there on the morning of admission. For a few days preceding admission, she had complained of feeling unwell, had a low-grade fever, and had spent most of her time resting in bed. Her participation in group activities in the nursing home had declined noticeably in the preceding days.

PMHx: Diabetes mellitus, chronic renal insufficiency, diabetic retinopathy, HTN

Meds: Glucophage, atenolol, enalapril

All: Sulfonamides

PE: Gen/CV: soft ejection systolic murmur. Lungs: decreased air entry left lung base

VS: Temp 100°F 100°C BP 165/95 HR 70

Neuro: Eyes closed, unarousable even to painful tactile stimuli. Pupils equally reactive. Normal oculocephalic reflexes. Gags when oropharynx suctioned.

Motor: No response to painful stimulation

Reflexes: Diffusely hyporeflexic, plantar response extensor

THOUGHT QUESTION

■ How will you categorize her condition?

Alteration in the level of consciousness is a common presentation in ED settings. The term encephalopathy is a nonspecific word used to indicate depression of level of awareness. Various states of abnormal mental function are recognized and it is important to be able to differentiate one from the other so as to make a diagnosis, identify the etiology, treat, and prognosticate.

Obtundation refers to a decreased level of awareness, from which a patient can be aroused by stimulation.

Stupor is a condition characterized by depression of level of consciousness from which a patient can be aroused, but requires stronger stimulation.

Coma is a condition of decreased level of consciousness, characterized by a lack of responsiveness to external stimulation or internal cues. The patient's eyes are closed, and the patient is unarousable even by noxious, vigorous stimulation.

Delirium refers to an abnormal mental state characterized by confusion, disorientation, and hallucinations (usually visual). Patients may be delirious intermittently, and periods of relative normalcy (lucency) may intersperse the delirium. Delirium is an acute, abnormal mental state, usually caused by some toxic-metabolic derangement that affects global cerebral function. Dementia is also an abnormal mental state that is characterized by a progressive, more or less permanent decline in cognitive function, without a change in level of arousal.

In the given clinical setting, the patient is unresponsive and unarousable even to repeated, vigorous, noxious stimulation. She does not flinch or wince when blood is drawn or an IV is placed. Her eyes are closed. Her state is consistent with coma.

CASE CONTINUED

Labs: CBC: Hb 9.7 g/dL, WBC: 16,000/mm³, 68% neutrophils, Plts: 150,000/mm³. Chemistries: electrolytes: WNL, glucose 250 mg/dL, BUN: 83 mg/dL, creatinine 6.3 mg/dL. LFTs: WNL. CSF: normal (Table 26-1).

TABLE 26-1 Common Causes of Coma

Infections	Endocrine	Head Trauma
Meningitis	Hypothyroidism (myxedema)	Postseizure
Encephalitis	Addisonian crisis	Inflammatory/ immunologic

Toxic/Metabolic	Focal CNS Lesions	Post-infectious Syndromes
Hypoxic-ischemic encephalopathy	Tumor	Connective tissue disorders
Hypoglycemia	Abscess	Granulomatous diseases
Hyperglycemia	Vascular	
Electrolyte abnormalities	Stroke	
Hepatic encephalopathy	Subarachnoid hemorrhage	
Uremic encephalopathy	Subdural/epidural hematoma	
Drug overdose	Cortical vein thrombosis	
Alcohol intoxication		

Imaging: Chest radiograph: Left lower-lobe pneumonia. Head CT: periventricular white matter disease (suggests chronic ischemic changes), old lacunar stroke in left internal capsule.

The patient is admitted and put on IV antibiotics. She is intubated for airway protection. Hemodialysis is also undertaken. Over the next 48 to 72 hours, her creatinine drops to 2.1, which is "baseline" for her. Her white count starts trending downward.

Her examination shows an improved mental status. Although still lethargic, she rouses to vigorous stimulation and is able to say her name. She moves all extremities to stimulation and her cranial nerve examination is normal. She is extubated 72 hours later.

It is learned from her nursing home that she had missed her chronic dialysis for several turns.

THOUGHT QUESTIONS

- How would you describe her state now?
- What is the likely etiology of her coma?

The patient now fits the description of stupor or obtundation. Her mental status is still abnormal, but improved.

The likely etiology of her coma is a toxic-metabolic encephalopathy from renal failure and an acute infection (pneumonia). Correction of the infection and metabolic abnormalities produced improvement in her condition.

QUESTIONS

26-1. A lesion in the midbrain will produce the following type of pupillary abnormality:
   A. Dilated pupils
   B. Midsized reactive pupils
   C. Pinpoint pupils
   D. Hyperactive hippus
   E. Argyll-Robertson pupils

26-2. A patient who appears comatose and has quadriparesis, facial weakness, and absent lateral eye movements (i.e., only vertical eye movements retained) is said to be:
   A. Vegetative
   B. Brain dead
   C. Locked in
   D. Stuporous
   E. Malingering

26-3. Patients in a vegetative state demonstrate:
   A. Limited ability to care for themselves
   B. Normal responsiveness
   C. Absence of brainstem reflexes
   D. Sleep/wake cycles
   E. All of the above

26-4. Which of the following are signs of raised intracranial pressure?
   A. Vomiting
   B. Papilledema
   C. HTN
   D. Bradycardia
   E. All of the above

ANSWERS

26-1. B. Typically midbrain lesions produce midsized reactive pupils. Pinpoint pupils are produced by pontine lesions. Argyll-Robertson pupils are pupils that constrict to accommodation but not to light. Dilated pupils are seen in a variety of conditions, e.g., sympathetic pathway lesions and oculomotor nerve lesions.

26-2. C. The situation described in the question is classic for a locked-in state classically seen in pontine lesions. The lesion disrupts corticospinal and corticobulbar pathways, leading to quadriparesis and inability to speak. The pathways responsible for wakefulness and arousal are spared, so the patient is not in a coma, but can communicate by moving his or her eyes in the vertical plane.

26-3. D. A patient in a vegetative state is not responsive, has intact brainstem reflexes, and demonstrates sleep/wake cycles. Vegetative state that persists beyond four weeks is termed "persistent vegetative state," from which the likelihood of a meaningful neurologic recovery is small.

26-4. E. Vomiting is a nonspecific sign of raised intracranial pressure. Papilledema (edema of the optic nerve head) is also a sign of raised intracranial pressure. HTN as a result of increased pressure occurs as part of the Cushing triad of HTN, bradycardia, and hyperventilation.

ADDITIONAL SUGGESTED READING

Baumgartner H, Gerstenbrand F. Diagnosing brain death without a neurologist. BMJ 2002;324:1471.

Saposnik G, Bueri JA, Maurino J, et al. Spontaneous and reflex movement in brain death. Neurology 2000;54:221.

V

Patients Who Present with Present with Hemiparesis and Generalized Weakness

CASE **27**

Acute Left-Sided Weakness

ID/CC: 68-year-old woman presents with acute onset of left-sided weakness.

HPI: Patient awoke unable to get out of bed, called for her husband who found her confused and unable to move her left side. She was in her usual state of good health when going to bed the night before.

PMHx: Osteoarthritis

PSHx: None

Meds: Ibuprofen

All: NKDA

SHx: Smokes three cigarettes a day for 40 years. Moderate alcohol consumption. Plays tennis five times a week.

FHx: Mother died of a skin disease. No history of CVAs.

Neuro Hx: None

THOUGHT QUESTIONS

- Where could her lesion(s) localize?
- What are other common findings in nondominant hemispheric lesions?
- Discuss the different etiologies and leading risk factors of stroke.

A left-sided hemiplegia can result from lesions of the left cervical spinal cord or the right brainstem, thalamus, internal capsule, or frontoparietal lobe.

The nondominant hemisphere in most people is on the right, with the exception a small number of left-handed individuals. The most obvious and dramatic signs of a large, nondominant hemispheric lesion is therefore, a left hemiparesis and left hemisensory loss. Because language function is by definition located in the dominant hemisphere, functional assessment of the nondominant hemisphere focuses primarily on other integrative tasks. Common symptoms of a nondominant hemispheric lesion include: (1) denial or lack of concern for functional deficits such as a hemiparesis; (2) left-sided neglect—the inability to recognize the left side of the world, often including their own body parts and inability to "see" people standing on their left or read the left face of a clock; (3) prosody (without melody) of speech—the patient's speech lacks the normal emotional inflections of speech often, even when conveying very upsetting news (monotonous) and often the patient cannot interpret the emotional content of the speech of others; (4) motor impersistence such as tongue protrusion; (5) spatial disorientation—the patient is unable to find his/her way around, often even in very familiar surroundings; (6) constructional apraxias—the patient is unable to copy simple diagrams and figures such as cubes; and (7) dressing apraxia—the patient no longer remembers how to put on his/her clothes.

Strokes or CVAs can be caused by disorders that result in the following: (1) local thrombosis of a cerebral vessel (atherosclerosis, hypercoagulable states); (2) emboli to the cerebral vasculature (artery-to-artery usually from atherosclerosis or cardiac emboli, often following a myocardial infarction or arrhythmia); (3) rupture of a cerebral vessel with consequent intracerebral hemorrhage (such as from uncontrolled HTN, ruptured vascular malformations, and amyloid deposits); (4) lacunar infarctions—small, often subclinical infarcts caused by local atherosclerosis or lipohyalinosis of small arterioles, usually in patients with long-standing diabetes mellitus or HTN (the most common clinically apparent lacunar strokes occur in the internal capsule, thalamus, basal ganglia, and brainstem); and (5) much less commonly, vasculitis, the inflammation of cerebral blood vessels most often because of infections, systemic vasculitides, and rarely, primary CNS vasculitis.

Stroke risk factors can be divided into two main groups; nonmodifiable and modifiable ones. Nonmodifiable ones include advanced age, male gender, Asian or African-American descent, and a family history of stroke. Modifiable risk factors include arterial HTN, systemic atherosclerotic disease (cardiac or other territories), diabetes mellitus, TIA, cigarette smoking, alcohol consumption, obesity, oral contraceptive use, and prior stroke (Fig. 27-1).

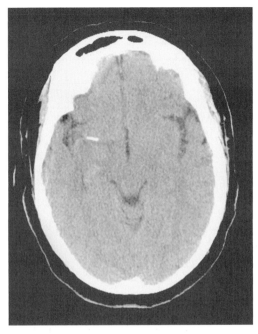

FIGURE 27-1
Head CT scan without contrast. (*Image courtesy of Dr. Ross Goldstein, Stanford University Medical Center, Stanford, California.*)

 CASE CONTINUED

VS: Temp 98.6°F BP 190/100 HR 76 RR 16

PE: Gen: Head and gaze deviated to right

Neuro: MSE: patient is confused and disoriented to place and time. Speech is monotone with no aphasia.

CN II–XII: Left-sided lower facial droop, diminished gag, otherwise intact

Motor: 0/5 strength left arm and leg with increased tone. Right-sided strength 5/5 with normal tone.

Reflexes: 3+ left arm and leg, 2+ right arm and leg. Babinski sign present on left.

Sensory: Patient does not respond to any stimuli on left. When shown her left hand she denies that it is part of her body.

Coordination: No tremor or nystagmus

Gait: Not testable

QUESTIONS

27-1. What artery supplies the territory of her infarction?
  A. Left vertebral
  B. Right vertebral
  C. Right recurrent artery of Heubner
  D. Right middle cerebral artery
  E. Right anterior cerebral artery

27-2. Her CT scan shows a large hypointense lesion in the right frontotemporoparietal lobe in the distribution of the middle cerebral artery with significant edema and midline shift. Which of the following is an appropriate treatment?
  A. IV heparin
  B. Antihypertensive treatment
  C. IV 5% dextrose-water
  D. Corticosteroids
  E. Mannitol

27-3. Which of the following additional work-up is most urgent?
  A. Carotid ultrasound
  B. Cardiac ECHO
  C. Hypercoagulable work-up (protein C, S, antithrombin III, factor V Leiden, serum homocysteine, antiphospholipid antibodies)
  D. ECG

27-4. Suppose the patient is a 38-year-old. What additional work-up should be done?
  A. Hypercoagulable work-up
  B. ANA, FTA, ESR
  C. Cerebrovascular angiogram
  D. Serum cholesterol, triglycerides, LDL, HDL profile
  E. All of the above

ANSWERS

27-1. D. A dense, left-sided hemiplegia, with left-sided neglect, lack of normal prosody of speech, and confusion is the classic presentation for a right middle cerebral artery infarct. This artery supplies the right posterior frontal lobe, right parietal lobe, and right anterior temporal lobe.

27-2. E. None of the above. The CT scan shows a very large infarct, therefore the risk of hemorrhagic conversion with the use of anticoagulants or thrombolytic agents such as heparin or tissue Plasminogen activator (t-PA) are unacceptable. The scan also shows evidence of edema, therefore fluids containing free water could dangerously increase the amount of cerebral edema and may be life-threatening. Corticosteroids have no role in treatment of cerebral edema as a result of strokes. Her HTN is the result of a normal reflex following strokes to increase the amount of cerebral blood flow. Rapid correction of HTN within the first 10 days following a stroke can lead to an extension of the stroke and should not be done unless it is critically high (diastolic persistently over 120 mm Hg). The appropriate treatments at this time are fluid restriction to minimize cerebral edema, aspiration, and deep vein thrombosis (DVT) prophylaxis, and careful neurologic monitoring for signs of herniation. Mannitol can be helpful in reducing the cytotoxic edema caused by large strokes.

27-3. D. The work-up in an elderly patient with a completed, large right MCA stroke should include a search for an embolic source (cardiac or artery-to-artery), evidence of a recent MI, and signs of a large-vessel arteritis (such as giant cell arteritis). The most urgent underlying cause to evaluate is a myocardial infarction. Hypercoagulable states are important causes of stroke in young people but not in the elderly.

27-4. E. In addition to the normal work-up for the source of an anterior circulation stroke because of cerebral infarction done in the elderly (CT scan, carotid Dopplers, cardiac ECHO, and a FANA, ESR, FTA, and CBC) important etiologies of stroke in the young include hypercoagulable states, vasculitis (reason for the cerebral angiogram), and inheritable disorders of lipid metabolism leading to premature atherosclerosis.

 ADDITIONAL SUGGESTED READING

Flemming KD, Brown RD Jr, Petty GW, et al. Evaluation and management of transient ischemic attack and minor cerebral infarction. Mayo Clin Proc 2004;79:1071.

Schneider AT, Kissela B, Woo D, et al. Ischemic stroke subtypes: a population-based study of incidence rates among blacks and whites. Stroke 2004;35:1552.

Worsening Left-Sided Weakness

ID/CC: 39-year-old woman who presents with left hemiplegia

HPI: MB is a 39-year-old woman who presented with a 1-day history of left arm numbness and weakness. Her symptoms progressed over the course of the day to left hemiplegia.

PMHx: Left arm deep venous thrombosis (DVT)

PSHx: None

Meds: Warfarin sodium (Coumadin)—noncompliant

All: NKDA

FHx: Mother with a history of CVA

Habits: No tobacco, no alcohol

VS: Temperature 96°F HR 81 BP 137/89 RR 18 SaO$_2$ 98% RA

PE/Neuro: The patient is an obese woman who is somnolent. She is arousable by sternal rub. She was not able to speak. She was able to follow simple commands. PERRL, she had a right gaze preference and a left visual field defect. The patient also had a right upper motor neuron facial droop. Her motor examination noted spontaneous movement in the right upper and lower extremities. She had a left hemiplegia.

THOUGHT QUESTION

- What is the differential diagnosis?

A thorough physical and neurologic examination is important. The patient's hemiplegia presenting initially as numbness and evolving to weakness is a key component of the history. Also the patient's history of DVT is significant in formulating a differential diagnosis. The primary concern is thus the possibility of a cerebrovascular event. Additionally, one must consider the possibility of an intracranial hemorrhage. This diagnosis is noted as the patient is on warfarin sodium (Coumadin) and the clinical presentation of a CVA and an intracranial hemorrhage can be the same.

CASE CONTINUED

A head CT and computed tomography angiography were obtained. It demonstrated a right MCA infarct and a left transverse sinus thrombosis. The patient was admitted to the ICU. Labs were obtained.

Labs: Comprehensive Metabolic Panel—WNL Coags—WNL

The patient was placed on a heparin drip and aggressive medical management was initiated. The patient remained stable for approximately 48 hours with improvement in level of consciousness. She was more awake and alert and continued to follow commands. On hospital day two she became unresponsive. She did not open her eyes. She remained nonverbal. Her pupils were dilated and unresponsive. She was unable to follow commands.

THOUGHT QUESTIONS

- What is the differential diagnosis?
- What is the next step in management?

 The patient was placed on heparin on admission. This raises the concern for a hemorrhagic evolution on the previously noted infarct. Other concerns include cerebral edema and increased intracranial pressure secondary to the evolution of the noted infarct.

Given the patient's decline in level of consciousness, the next step is to ensure protection of her airway, i.e., intubation, and to try to address the clinical presentation of raised intracranial pressure.

CASE CONTINUED

She was intubated for airway protection. Additionally, she was treated with hyperosmolar therapy and transient hyperventilation. Additionally, an emergent head CT scan was obtained. The scan demonstrated an evolution of the previously noted infarct with subfalcine and uncal herniation. The basal cisterns were also effaced. The neurosurgery team was contacted for possible intervention. The patient's pupils returned to normal size and became responsive following the above maneuvers.

CT SCAN—Evolution of large right MCA infarct resulting in subfalcine and uncal herniation with effacement of the basilar cisterns. There is significant mass effect with associated midline shift. There is no hemorrhagic transformation noted.

In review of all available options, the decision was made for surgical intervention. She was taken to the operating room and underwent a decompressive craniectomy with augmentation duraplasty. There were no intra-operative complications. The patient tolerated the procedure.

The patient returned to the ICU. She improved neurologically and was extubated on post op day three. She was awake and alert and able to follow simple commands with a persisting left hemiplegia. She received physical, occupational, and speech therapy and was discharged to a rehabilitation facility.

QUESTIONS

28-1. Which of the following is used in the first-tier management of raised intracranial pressure?
  A. Hypothermia
  B. Mild hyperventilation
  C. Decompressive craniectomy
  D. Induced HTN

28-2. Which of the following is used in the second-tier management of raised intracranial pressure?

    A. Osmotic diuresis

    B. Mild to moderate hyperventilation

    C. Induced HTN

    D. All of the above

28-3. In the setting of ischemic stroke, patients suffer which of the following?

    A. Cytotoxic edema only

    B. Vasogenic edema only

    C. Both cytotoxic and vasogenic edema

    D. Neither cytotoxic nor vasogenic edema

28-4. The middle cerebral artery and its various branches supply all but which of the following?

    A. Uncus

    B. Optic chiasm

    C. Superior parietal lobule

    D. Supply all of the above

ANSWERS

28-1. B. Mild to moderate hyperventilation is a first tier management. Aggressive hyperventilation is a second-tier management tool. All other listed treatments are considered second-tier management options.

28-2. C. Induced HTN is considered a second-tier management option. All other listed treatments are considered first-tier management options.

28-3. C. Patients who have suffered ischemic strokes sustain both cytotoxic and vasogenic edema. The onset of cytotoxic edema is variable, but usually within hours of the onset of the stroke.

28-4. C. The anterior cerebral artery supplies the optic chiasm.

ADDITIONAL SUGGESTED READING

Mori K, Nakao Y, Yamamoto T, et al. Early external decompressive craniectomy with duroplasty improves functional recovery in patients with massive hemispheric embolic infarction

timing and indication of decompressive surgery for malignant
cerebral infarction. Surg Neurol 2004;62:420–430.

Robertson SC, Lennarson P, Hasan DM, et al. Clinical course and
surgical management of massive cerebral infarction.
Neurosurgery 2004;55:55–62.

Winter CD, Adamides AA, Rosenfeld JV. The role of decompressive
craniectomy in the management of traumatic brain injury:
a critical review. J Clin Neuro 2005;12:619–623.

Hemiparesis Following Trauma

ID/CC: 27-year-old man involved in a motor vehicle accident who presents with right hemiparesis

HPI: HI, a helmeted driver of a motorcycle, was struck by an automobile traveling at approximately 55 mph. Initially Mr. I was alert and oriented. He had multiple abrasions and a scalp laceration and complained of mild neck pain. En route to the hospital, via paramedics, the patient's level of consciousness began to decline and he became more difficult to arouse. He was brought to the emergency room for further evaluation.

PMHx: None

PSHx: None

Meds: None

Allergies: NKDA

SHx: The patient is single and lives alone.

Habits: No tobacco, occasional alcohol, no IVDA or recreational drugs

VS: Temp 98.9°F BP 125/84 HR 88 RR 14

PE/Neuro: There are multiple abrasions of the head and neck. There is a small laceration on the left forehead. The patient opens eyes to verbal command. He is oriented to person, place, and time, and follows simple commands.

There is mild weakness noted in the right upper and lower extremities, 4/5.

There is reflex asymmetry with the right patellar reflex 3. An extensor plantar response is present on the right (Babinski reflex).

Labs: All WNL

Imaging: Cervical spine radiograph: no fractures, normal alignment, no evidence of soft tissue damage

THOUGHT QUESTIONS

- Where would you localize the lesion and what is the differential diagnosis? What is the significance of the Babinski reflex?
- What scoring system would be used to evaluate the patient's level of consciousness?
- What test is the most important in confirming a diagnosis at this stage?

The patient's differential diagnosis includes epidural hematoma and subdural hematoma. Both of these diagnoses are associated with significant morbidity and mortality and may require emergent surgical intervention (see discussion below for more detail). The plantar reflex known as the Babinski sign is a primitive reflex present in infancy and disappears usually by the first year of life. An upper motor neuron lesion anywhere from the pyramidal tract to L4 can result in an abnormal reflex, i.e., extension of the big toe.

The Glasgow coma scale (GCS) is a scoring system used to assess level of consciousness. It assesses three main categories: eyes, best motor response, and best verbal response. The scale ranges from 3 (worst response) to 15 (best score). See question 29-1 for details.

Given the patient is hemodynamically stable, an emergent noncontrast head computed tomography (CT) is the most important diagnostic test at this stage. The CT scan can identify the presence of acute blood and associated fractures. Additionally, the CT scan is essential in formulating a treatment plan and will aid in surgical planning.

CASE CONTINUED

While preparing for transfer to CT scan, the patient becomes progressively less responsive. He opens his eyes only to painful stimuli and although still able to talk, he is disoriented. He moves bilateral upper extremities to painful stimuli only and then demonstrates flexion withdrawal. In addition, his pupils are asymmetric with the right at 6 mm and the left at 4 mm.

CT Scan: Noncontrast CT demonstrates a large 2.5-cm biconvex hyperdense acute left temporoparietal hematoma (Fig. 29-1).

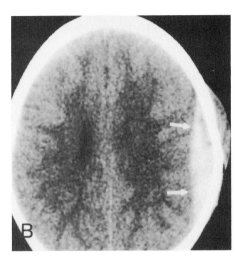

FIGURE 29-1
Intracranial manifestations of head injury. Epidural bleed (arrows) with some soft-tissue swelling of the scalp. (*From Swischuk LE. Emergency imaging of the acutely ill or injured child, 3rd Ed. Philadelphia: Lippincott, Williams & Wilkins, 1994:595.*)

The patient is brought emergently to the operating room where a craniotomy is performed for evacuation of an epidural hematoma. The source of the bleeding was identified and coagulated.

 QUESTIONS

29-1. What is the initial GCS of the patient in the ED?
A. 15
B. 14
C. 10
D. 17

29-2. What is the most likely source of the epidural hematoma?
A. Tearing of bridging veins
B. Laceration of venous sinuses
C. Laceration of the middle meningeal artery
D. None of the above

29-3. What percent of epidural hematomas are associated with fractures?
- A. 10%
- B. 25%
- C. 50%
- D. 85%

29-4. What is the overall mortality rate of epidural hematoma?
- A. 5%
- B. 25%
- C. 50%
- D. 75%

 ANSWERS

29-1. B. The ED evaluation of the patient yields a GCS of 14: eyes (3)—opens to verbal command, motor (6)—obeys and follows command, verbal (5)—oriented to person, place, and time. The following table provides details regarding scoring for the GCS. The maximum score (normal) is 15, the worst score (most severe coma) is 3 (Table 29-1).

TABLE **29-1**   The Glasgow Coma Scale

Points	Best Eye Opening	Best Verbal	Best Motor
1	None	None	None
2	To pain	Incomprehensible	Extensor
3	To speech	Inappropriate	Flexion
4	Spontaneous	Confused	Withdraws to pain
5		Oriented	Localizes to pain
6			Obeys

Teasdale G, Jennett B. Assessment of Coma and Impaired Consciousness: a Practical Scale. Lancet 1974;2:81–4.

29-2. C. The most likely source of hemorrhage in an epidural hematoma is a laceration of the middle meningeal artery. Other common sources are from a dural sinus or a diploic vein. Tearing of the bridging veins is associated with subdural hematomas.

29-3. D. Fractures are frequently associated with epidural hematomas. Approximately 85% of epidural hematomas are associated with skull fractures. The traditional teaching poses two mechanisms for the formation of epidural hematomas. One theory holds that the temporoparietal skull fracture is the primary event that ruptures the middle meningeal artery. This causes arterial bleeding that separates the dura from the inner table of the skull, and blood collects in the space. The second theory holds that separation of the dura is the primary event, forming a potential space into which bleeding occurs.

The classic presentation of an epidural hematoma occurs in a minority of affected patients. These patients present with a brief loss of consciousness, followed by a lucid interval, and then by obtundation, contralateral hemiparesis, and ipsilateral papillary dilation. Other more frequent presentation includes headache, vomiting, and seizures.

29-4. A. The overall mortality rate of epidural hematomas is 5%.

 ## ADDITIONAL SUGGESTED READING

Saito T, Kushi H, Makino K, et al. The risk factors for the occurrence of acute brain swelling in acute subdural hematoma. Acta Neurochir Suppl 2003;86:351–354.

Progressive Hemiparesis

ID/CC: 72-year-old man who presents with complaint of progressive right-sided weakness over 2 weeks

HPI: Two weeks prior to presentation, PH tripped and fell while playing tennis. There was no loss of consciousness and no associated injuries noted. Since then, he has developed increasing difficulties using his left upper extremity and weakness in his left leg. He has also had headaches increasing in both frequency and intensity. He was brought to the ED by his wife, who has noticed his increasing weakness.

PMHx: BPH, Hx of melanoma

PSHx: s/p resection of melanoma 5 years ago

Meds: None

Allergies: PCN

SHx: Married with four adult children. Lives at home with his wife. Retired engineer.

Habits: No tobacco, glass of wine every evening, no IVDA or recreational drugs

VS: Temp 98.1°F BP 136/85 HR 92 RR 16

PE/Neuro: The patient was alert and oriented to person, place, and time. CNs are intact. He has healing ecchymosis on the right forearm and thigh. There is increased tone in the left upper extremity. There are no associated muscle fasciculations or muscle wasting. Pronator drift is noted on the left side. Weakness (4/5) is noted in all motor groups of the left upper extremity. Reflexes are brisk and symmetric throughout the upper and lower extremities with the exception of an extensor plantar response on the left.

Labs: Hematocrit 33

Imaging studies: CT head: (Fig. 30-1)

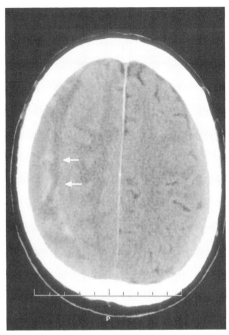

FIGURE **30-1**
A noncontrast CT was obtained that demonstrated mixed density (isodense and hyperdense) extra-axial concave hematomas in the right and left fronto-parietal regions. The collection is largest on the right, measuring 2 cm, versus 1 cm on the left. These findings are consistent with subdural hematoma. (*Image provided by the Departments of Neuroradiology and Neurosurgery, Stanford University, Stanford, California.*)

THOUGHT QUESTIONS

- Is the patient's examination consistent with an upper or lower motor neuron lesion?
- What is the patient's differential diagnosis?
- Would you obtain a noncontrast or contrast head CT?

PH's neurologic examination is consistent with an upper motor neuron lesion. Specifically, the examination demonstrates involvement of both the upper and lower extremities and an abnormal Babinski reflex.

Given the patient's history of melanoma, the differential diagnosis must include metastatic brain tumor. Given the recent history of trauma, post-traumatic subdural hematoma must also be considered.

In order to evaluate for the presence of extra-axial blood, a noncontrast head CT should be obtained first. Should this evaluation be negative, proceed to a contrast study in order to better assess for the presence of metastatic lesion(s).

 CASE CONTINUED

A noncontrast CT was obtained that demonstrated mixed density (isodense and hyperdense) extra-axial concave hematomas in the right and left frontoparietal regions. The collection is largest on the right, measuring 2 cm versus 1 cm on the left.

These findings are consistent with subdural hematoma.

After discussing the risks and benefits of available treatment options, the decision was made to undergo surgical evacuation of the hematoma.

 QUESTIONS

30-1. Which of the following metastatic tumors is the most likely to hemorrhage?
- A. Lung
- B. Melanoma
- C. Breast
- D. Prostate

30-2. What is the overall mortality rate of subdural hematomas?
- A. <5%
- B. 10% to 25%
- C. >60%
- D. 30%

30-3. What is the most likely source of the subdural hematoma?
- A. Tearing of bridging veins
- B. Laceration of venous sinuses
- C. Laceration of the middle meningeal artery
- D. None of the above

30-4. In the management of both subdural hematomas and metastatic lesions which of the following modalities might be utilized?
   A. Anticonvulsants
   B. Whole brain radiation therapy
   C. Anticoagulation
   D. All of the above

 ANSWERS

30-1. D. Although melanomas are a relatively rare cancer, they are a frequent source of intracranial metastases. Additionally, they are among the most frequent metastases to hemorrhage. Other common hemorrhagic metastatic tumors are choriocarcinoma and renal cell carcinoma. The most common primary tumors that spread to brain are lung and breast cancer.

30-2. C. The mortality rate of subdural hematomas far exceeds that of epidural hematomas. The overall mortality rate is estimated to be between 60% and 90%.

30-3. A. The most likely source of subdural hematomas is tearing of bridging veins. Laceration of middle meningeal artery and/or laceration of venous sinuses are common sources of epidural hematomas.

30-4. A. Seizures are a common presentation of metastatic disease. Seizures are also a frequent occurrence in patients with subdural hematomas. Anticonvulsants are used in the management of both cerebral metastases and subdural hematomas. The routine use of anticonvulsants in the setting of post-traumatic seizures remains controversial. WBRT is not a treatment modality utilized in the management of subdural hematomas. The use of anticoagulation is contraindicated in both subdural hematomas and cerebral metastases. A noted exception is the concomitant diagnosis of Trousseau's syndrome, which is a hypercoagulable state presenting in the setting of malignancy.

 ADDITIONAL SUGGESTED READING

de Gans J, van de Beek D. Dexamethasone in adults with bacterial meningitis. N Engl J Med 2002;347:1549.
Hasbun R, Abrahams J, Jekel J, et al. Computed tomography of the head before LP in adults with suspected meningitis. N Engl J Med 2001;345:1727.

Generalized Weakness in an Adult

ID/CC: 58-year-old man presents with worsening generalized weakness over the last 4 months.

HPI: TS first noticed the onset of weakness in his legs 4 months ago. He would stumble on occasion and then developed difficulty arising out of a chair. Soon thereafter, he began dropping things and having difficulty putting away dishes or other objects in higher cabinets. On neurologic review of systems he has stocking-glove distribution numbness and tingling for 2 months but no pain. He denies any orthostatic lightheadedness, fainting spells, reduced or excessive sweating, or change in bladder, bowel, or sexual function. No anorexia, early satiety, or nausea (gastroparesis). No muscle cramps or change in gait or balance. No trouble swallowing or slurred speech. There is no diurnal variation to his symptoms.

PMHx: HTN

PSHx: None

Meds: Atenolol 50 mg by mouth four times a day

All: NKDA

SHx: Salesman, no alcohol or tobacco use. Divorced.

FHx: No history of neurologic illnesses or difficulty walking

VS: 98.6°F BP 130/70 HR 76 Orthostatics WNL

PE: Unremarkable

Neuro: Notable for the following:

Motor: Muscle strength (out of 5) as follows: deltoids 3, biceps 4, triceps 5, wrist flexors and extensors 5, intrinsic hand muscles 3; iliopsoas 3, knee extensors and flexors 5, plantar and dorsiflexion, ankle eversion 3, ankle inversion 5. Mild muscular wasting in the bilateral deltoid muscles. Tone is slightly diminished in the lower extremities, normal elsewhere.

Reflexes: Absent throughout

Sensory: Diminished to light touch in a symmetrical, stocking-glove distribution. Slight decrease to vibration and joint position sense in the bilateral toes.

THOUGHT QUESTIONS

- How would you summarize the case thus far?
- Discuss the general approach to evaluating a patient with a peripheral neuropathy.

A 58-year-old man with no family history of neurologic illness presents with subacute, progressive weakness affecting all four extremities, involving proximal and distal strength equally. He is areflexic and has stocking-glove distribution numbness. Bulbar, autonomic, and cerebellar function appear intact. Based on his history and PE he most likely has a peripheral polyneuropathy.

When evaluating a patient with a possible neuropathy one must first establish by history and PE whether it involves an isolated peripheral nerve (mononeuropathy), several discrete individual nerves (multifocal mononeuropathy), or is a process affecting peripheral nerves diffusely (polyneuropathy). The distribution of weakness and sensory changes and the extent of autonomic involvement affect the differential diagnosis. Peripheral polyneuropathies are usually symmetrical and are more pronounced in the lower extremities. Many polyneuropathies begin distally and only much later in the course involve proximal muscles; however, this is not always the case as in this patient. Next, it is important to try to distinguish whether the disease process is more likely producing axonal damage, demyelination, or both. While the NCV and to a lesser extent the EMG is the best way to distinguish these, there are important clinical clues. Axonal peripheral neuropathies are the most common form of peripheral neuropathy and are usually because of systemic metabolic disorders or toxins and, less commonly, to hereditary disorders (hereditary motor-sensory neuropathy [HMSN] type II). Clinically, it presents with symmetrical, distal sensory and motor dysfunction starting in the legs, extending proximally in a graded fashion. Loss of reflexes and muscle atrophy are usually in proportion to the degree of weakness (e.g. stocking-glove distribution numbness, symmetrical weakness of dorsi- and plantar flexion with atrophy and loss of ankle jerks). Demyelinating peripheral neuropathies are usually because of immune-mediated damage of the myelin sheath or hereditary disorders (HMSN IA and III, Refsum disease, and leukodystrophies). Clinical clues are weakness out of proportion to the degree of atrophy, equal degree of weakness in proximal and distal muscle groups, early loss of all reflexes, and the presence of tremor or palpably enlarged nerves.

 CASE CONTINUED

Labs: EMG/NCV: reduction of motor conduction velocities below 70% of normal with areas of conduction block in multiple motor nerves, and absent F-waves.

CSF: WBC 1, RBC 0, protein 100 mg/dL, glucose WNL

Sural-nerve
biopsy: Moderate reduction of large myelinated fibers with areas of endoneurial mononuclear inflammatory infiltrates.

 QUESTIONS

31-1. The history, exam, CSF findings, and EMG/NCV are suggestive of which disorder?
   A. Axonal polyneuropathy because of primary biliary cirrhosis
   B. Demyelinating polyneuropathy because of CIDP
   C. Axonal polyneuropathy because of diabetes
   D. All of the above

31-2. What additional work-up should be done?
   A. FANA, ESR, manual peripheral blood smear, and HIV testing
   B. FANA, ESR, manual peripheral blood smear, and porphyrin screen
   C. FANA, ESR, manual peripheral blood smear, and heavy metal screen
   D. HIV testing, porphyrin, and heavy metal screen

31-3. Suppose the additional work-up is negative. What is the most likely diagnosis?
   A. Guillain-Barré's syndrome (GBS)
   B. CIDP
   C. Hereditary leukodystrophy
   D. Amyloid neuropathy

31-4. Which of the following treatment options would be inappropriate in this patient?
   A. Plasma exchange
   B. High-dose prednisone
   C. IV immune globulin
   D. Azathioprine plus prednisone
   E. All of the above

ANSWERS

31-1. C. NCVs are the most useful test to distinguish between axonal and demyelinating peripheral neuropathies. In the case of axonal neuropathies (the axon is damaged but the myelin sheath is intact) there is a reduction in the amplitude of sensory nerve action potentials (SNAPs) and compound muscle action potentials (CMAPs), but the velocity of conduction is normal to only slightly impaired. In demyelinating neuropathies the myelin sheath is damaged and repaired usually in a segmental fashion, resulting in areas of abnormally thin myelin and with repeated damage, excessive proliferation of Schwann cells forming so-called onion bulbs. The end result is areas of marked slowing of the nerve conduction velocities (less than 70% of the lower limits of normal), mixed with conduction block, dispersion of CMAPs, and prolonged or absent latencies of distal and F-waves.

The history, examination, NCV, CSF (isolated elevated protein), and biopsy findings are all characteristic of an acquired demyelinating peripheral neuropathy. The most common causes of an acquired demyelinating peripheral neuropathy are dysproteinemias, osteosclerotic myeloma, and CIDP. Diabetes is associated with multifocal mononeuropathies, entrapment mononeuropathies (carpal tunnel syndrome), and axonal peripheral polyneuropathies.

31-2. A. This patient should be worked up for the above illnesses, which would include serum and urine protein electrophoresis and a skeletal bone survey. CIDP can be associated with HIV infection, chronic active hepatitis, inflammatory bowel disease, systemic lupus erythematosus, polyneuropathy, organomegaly, endocrinopathy, M protein, and skin changes (POEMS) syndrome, and Hodgkin lymphoma. Porphyria and heavy metal toxin-induced (lead, arsenic) neuropathies cause axonal neuropathies with distinctive clinical pictures.

31-3. B. Once associated systemic illnesses have been ruled out, the most likely diagnosis is idiopathic CIDP. This disorder occurs typically during the fifth and sixth decade, and is characterized clinically by a subacute/chronic progressive or relapsing course of muscle weakness for more than 2 months associated with areflexia.

31-4. E. In a patient with moderately severe CIDP as this patient has, the first-line treatment is either high-dose prednisone (80 mg/day for 4 weeks) or plasma exchange (two times a week for 4 weeks). If there were no improvement then the next choice would be either IV immune globulin or plasma exchange with high-dose prednisone.

 ADDITIONAL SUGGESTED READING

Argyriou AA, Chroni E, Koutras A, et al. Vitamin E for prophylaxis against chemotherapy-induced neuropathy: a randomized controlled trial. Neurology 2005;64:26.

Ferrante MA. Brachial plexopathies: classification, causes, and consequences. Muscle Nerve 2004;30:547.

Bilateral Foot Drop, Lower Extremity Numbness, and Tingling

ID/CC: Patient is a 26-year-old woman with new numbness, lower extremity weakness.

HPI: Patient is a 26-year-old right-handed woman who was well until 2 weeks ago. At that time, she had 2 days of diarrhea that resolved. At that time, she started to notice a tingling sensation in both her shins. She had no pain or numbness. Two days later, she noticed that she kept tripping on her right foot and felt that she had a more difficult time lifting it off the ground. She denies any bowel or bladder incontinence. Today, she has come to the emergency room because she is having some difficulty breathing. A neurology consult is called because of her previous symptoms.

PMHx: One prior pregnancy without any complications.

PSHx: Negative

Meds: Multivitamin

All: NKDA

FHx: Noncontributory

SHx: Works as an attorney. No history of smoking or alcohol use.

PE: Gen: Vital signs normal. Ophthalmologic examination completely normal including visual acuity and slit-lamp examination.

Neuro: Mental status: normal orientation and attention.

CN II–XII: Intact. Extra-ocular movements are full, pupils are equal and reactive without any afferent pupillary defect, visual fields are full, normal funduscopic examination.

**Motor
examination:**   Tone: normal. Strength 5/5 in right upper extremity, 4/5 in right dorsiflexion. 5/5 in left upper and lower extremities.

Reflexes: Absent reflexes at ankles and knees

Cerebellum: No dysmetria or ataxia

THOUGHT QUESTIONS

- Where can I localize this lesion?
- What work-up is indicated?
- How do I triage this patient?

When patients present with lower extremity weakness and sensory changes, without any mental status changes, cranial nerve palsies, or upper extremity symptoms, localization can be challenging because the entire length of the nervous system can be responsible. It is always helpful to evaluate negative symptoms such as numbness and weakness backwards from the end organ to the neuromuscular junction to the distal neuron to the proximal neuron to the brain. When patients present with bilateral symptoms, the localization can be narrowed significantly. With a few notable exceptions in the midline, such as a peri-falcine mengioma, a single lesion in the brain will usually cause lateralizing signs. Spinal cord lesions, because of the narrow geography, can often have bilateral symptoms. Peripheral nerves usually cause unilateral deficits as well unless the process is multifocal. PE findings such as muscle bulk, tone, and reflexes can be instrumental in helping you to determine if weakness is in an upper motor neuron or lower motor neuron distribution.

After the examination, appropriate imaging of the brain and spine is indicated. With bilateral motor and sensory symptoms, this patient should have an MRI of her entire spine. Evaluation of the spinal fluid can be helpful to determine if there is an inflammatory, infectious, or neoplastic process. Whenever there is a question of a patient's ability to ambulate, or if a patient has a new cardiac or respiratory complaint, admission to a closely observed setting is usually indicated.

This patient may have Guillain-Barré's syndrome, syndrome of an idiopathic inflammatory demyelinating polyneuropathy. Patients will often present with paresthesias in addition to weakness, back pain, and loss of reflexes. Respiratory weakness is a feared complication of this syndrome, and patients often need mechanical ventilation.

CASE CONTINUED

Lab: CBC: WNL-electrolytes, glucose, LFTs: WNL. CSF – 1 red blood cell, 3 white blood cells, protein 150, glucose 65. Gram stain negative

Imaging: MRI spine: No abnormalities or cord compression

QUESTIONS

32-1. Guillain-Barré can be treated by which of the following?
A. Prednisone
B. Ribavirin
C. Plasmapheresis
D. Sinemet
E. Doxycycline

32-2. Which of the following systemic complications can be seen as a direct result of Guillain-Barré?
A. Deep vein thrombosis
B. Sinusitis
C. Severe hypotension
D. Bacterial sepsis
E. Nephrotic's syndrome

32-3. Which of the following treatments has been associated with Guillain-Barré's syndrome?
A. Influenza vaccination
B. Oral contraceptive therapy
C. Antibiotic therapy
D. Steroids
E. Aspirin

32-4. Which of the following is an upper motor neuron sign?
A. Atrophy
B. Hyporeflexia
C. Downgoing toe
D. Clonus
E. Fasciculations

ANSWERS

32-1. C. IV immunoglobulin (IVIG) and plasmapheresis have both been used to treat Guillain-Barré. Several studies have compared the two therapies, and one has not been found to be more efficacious than the other. While logistical considerations often determine which therapy will be used, ideally, plasmapheresis is used before IVIG treatment so that the antibodies are not removed. Steroids have no proven benefit in this disorder.

32-2. C. Patients with Guillain-Barré may have significant dysautonomias including BP fluctuations and arrhythmias. Care must be taken when using any vasoactive medications. They can also have impaired control of bladder function and may have urinary tract infections as well.

32-3. A. There has been a rare, sporadic association in previous years between the influenza vaccine and Guillain-Barré. Other associations include Campylobacter jejuni, CMV, Epstein-Barr virus (EBV), HIV, and Lyme disease. Current recommendations suggest that patients who acquired the syndrome within 6 weeks of an influenza vaccination avoid using the vaccine in future years if they are at low risk for acquiring the virus.

32-4. D. Upper motor neuron signs include hyperreflexia, spasticity and increased tone, and an upgoing toe (or positive Babinski). Clonus is a series of repetitive, rhythmic contractions in a stretched state.

ADDITIONAL SUGGESTED READING

Brannagan TH 3rd, Zhou Y. HIV-associated Guillain-Barré's syndrome. J Neurol Sci 2003;208:39.
Haber P, DeStefano F, Angulo FJ, et al. Guillain-Barré's syndrome following influenza vaccination. JAMA 2004;292:2478.

Progressive Numbness and Weakness

ID/CC: 33-year-old man with a complaint of progressive numbness and weakness of his extremities.

HPI: JR presented with an 8-month history of progressive numbness and weakness. There was no antecedent event. Specifically, Mr. R denied any history of trauma. The symptoms began in the right hand and progressed to involve the left upper extremity and both lower extremities. The right-sided symptoms were worse than the left and the upper extremities were more involved than the lower extremities. There was no associated pain. JR denied any bowel or bladder symptoms, but he complained of penile numbness. He denied any other associated complaints.

PMHx: HTN

PSHx: None

Meds: None

SHx: The patient is married. He is unemployed.

Habits: The patient denied any alcohol, tobacco, or illicit drug use.

VS: WNL

PE: The general PE was without abnormalities. His neurologic examination noted upper extremity weakness.

Right Upper Extremity Motor Examination—deltoid—4/5, biceps—4/5, triceps—3/5, wrist flexors—3/5, wrist extensors—3/5.

Left Upper Extremity Motor Examination—deltoid—4/5, biceps—4/5, triceps—4/5, wrist flexors—4/5, wrist extensors—4/5.

Right Lower Extremity Motor Examination—All groups were 4 + /5.

Left Lower Extremity Motor Examination—All groups were 5/5.

Reflexes: Throughout. Hoffman's sign was positive on the right.

Sensory: Decreased sensation to light touch and pinprick throughout the right hemi body compared to the left.

Labs: WNL

THOUGHT QUESTIONS

- What is the differential diagnosis?
- What studies should be obtained?

The differential diagnosis includes neoplasm. Specifically, spinal cord tumors, which can be extradural, intradural-extramedullary, or intradural-intramedullary. Vascular lesions must also be considered and would include conditions such as arteriovenous malformations (AVMs). Other less common etiologies include autoimmune disorders such as multiple sclerosis (MS).

The next studies necessary are an MRI of the spine, routine laboratory studies, and Vitamin B and thyroid levels.

CASE CONTINUED

All laboratory and endocrine studies were WNL.

An MRI scan with and without contrast was obtained. It demonstrated an intramedullary spinal cord tumor eccentric to the right extending from C2–C7. There is associated edema and an associated syrinx (Fig. 33-1).

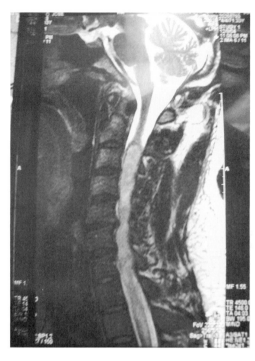

FIGURE 33-1
An MRI scan with and without contrast was obtained. It demonstrated an intramedullary spinal cord tumor eccentric to the right extending from C2–C7. There is associated edema and an associated syrinx. (*From Greenberg VM, Adams RD. Intraspinal Tumors. Principles of Neurology, 2nd Ed. New York: McGraw-Hill, 1981:638–641.*)

THOUGHT QUESTION

▪ What is your differential diagnosis at this time?

As the radiographs demonstrate that the lesion is an intramedullary tumor, the differential diagnosis can be narrowed. Intramedullary tumors include astrocytomas, ependymomas, dermoids, epidermoids, and multiple other miscellaneous lesions.

CASE CONTINUED

In review of the history, PE, radiographic findings, and all available treatment options, the decision was made for operative intervention. The patient was brought to the operating room by the neurosurgery team. He underwent multilevel cervical laminectomies with resection of the identified intramedullary tumor.

The procedure was performed with the assistance of electrophysiological monitoring. There were no intra-operative complications. The patient tolerated the procedure well. The postoperative neurologic examination was unchanged from the pre-operative examination.

QUESTIONS

33-1. What is the most common intramedullary spinal cord tumor outside of the filum terminale?
- A. Dermoid
- B. Epidermoid
- C. Astrocytoma
- D. Metastases

33-2. What is the most common glioma of the lower spinal cord, conus medullaris, and filum terminale?
- A. Astrocytoma
- B. Ependymoma
- C. Oligodendroglioma
- D. None of the above

33-3. What is the most common presenting complaint of spinal cord tumors?
- A. Pain
- B. Visible mass over the spine
- C. Paresthesias
- D. Weakness

33-4. Ependymomas do not express which of the following?
- A. Glial fibrillary acidic protein (GFAP)
- B. S100
- C. Vimentin
- D. Synaptophysin

ANSWERS

33-1. C. Astrocytomas are the most common intramedullary spinal cord tumor outside of the filum terminale.

33-2. B. Ependymoma is the most common glioma of the lower spinal cord, conus medullaris, and filum terminale.

33-3. A. Pain is the most common presenting complaint. Weakness is the second most common clinical complaint. The other symptoms listed are less frequently reported complaints.

33-4. D. The great majority of ependymomas display GFAP immunoreactivity. They typically express S100 protein and vimentin. Ependymomas do not express neuronal antigens such as synaptophysin.

 ADDITIONAL SUGGESTED READING

Adams RD, Victor M. Intraspinal tumors. Principles of Neurology, 2nd Ed. New York: McGraw-Hill, 1981:638–641.

Citow JS, Macdonald RL, Kraig RP, Wollmann RL. Comprehensive Neurosurgery Board Review. New York, NY: Thieme, 2000.

Greenberg MS. Handbook of Neurosurgery. New York, NY: Thieme, 2001:480–484.

Kleihues P, Cavenee WK. World Health Organization Classification of Tumors Pathology and Genetics Tumors of the Nervous System. Lyon (France): IARC Press, 2000:74, 115, 71, 55.

Floppy Infant

ID/CC: A 4-month-old infant presenting with weak arms and legs.

HPI: WH is a 4-month-old infant brought to his pediatrician for assessment of developmental delay. At 4 months his head control was poor. He did not lift his head off the pillow. When picked up, his head fell back as his neck was weak. He fed from a bottle, taking a long time to finish his feeds as his sucking was slow and weak.

On further questioning, the parents stated that he was always alert and made good eye contact. He began smiling at 6 weeks of age, and recognized his parents. He turned his eyes and head to sound and has begun to coo a little.

The child's mother was healthy during pregnancy. This was her second pregnancy, and she thought that this child was less active than her first baby. He was born at home, and delivery was uncomplicated. Birth-weight was 2.7 kg. The neonatal period was unremarkable.

PMHx: As above

Meds: Infant vitamin drops

All: None

FHx: Noncontributory

SHx: Second child. Older child is a 3-year-old boy, who is healthy.

PE: Gen: HEENT: not dysmorphic. CV: mild sinus tachycardia. Resp: Tachypneic, subcostal retraction. Lungs: Clear. No organomegaly.

VS: Afebrile. HR 136 RR 40. Weight: 4.4 kg, OFC: 42 cm (25th percentile)

Neuro: Mental status: alert, smiles and interacts with mom.

Cranial nerves: Normal.

Motor: Decreased muscle tone in axial and limb muscles. Head lag when pulled from supine to prone position. When supine, legs are in a "frog-leg" position.

Reflexes: Not elicitable. When the baby cries, ripples of muscle contraction can be seen on the tongue

THOUGHT QUESTIONS

- What is the primary problem?
- How will you localize the lesion?

The most striking feature in this case is hypotonia. Clues to hypotonia are reduced fetal movements, weak sucking, and key findings on neurologic examination (see questions below).

While evaluating an infant with hypotonia, one must begin with whether the hypotonia is from an upper motor neuron or lower motor neuron lesion. Features of an upper motor neuron process are: encephalopathy, delayed cognitive development, cranial nerve abnormalities, vision or hearing abnormalities, and normal/brisk deep tendon reflexes. Features suggestive of a lower motor neuron process are normal mentation, weakness out of proportion to the hypotonia, muscle atrophy/fasciculations, and hypoactive or absent deep tendon reflexes.

In this patient key features are profound hypotonia and weakness, absent reflexes, and normal mentation. This suggests a lower motor neuron lesion. In myopathies, proximal weakness is greater than distal weakness; in neuropathies the pattern of weakness is the opposite. The presence of abnormal eye movements, ptosis, and prominent feeding difficulties early on would suggest a neuromuscular junction abnormality. The profound weakness and hypotonia, lack of deep tendon reflexes, and tongue fasciculations (ripples on the tongue) are highly suggestive of an anterior horn cell disease.

While evaluating a neonate with hypotonia, often making an accurate localization along the neuraxis can be difficult. Once it is established that one is dealing with a lower motor neuron lesion, the usual work-up consists of checking muscle enzymes (creatine phosphokinase [CPK], aspartate aminotransferase [AST]). Sometimes an EMG/ nerve conduction study is obtained, but these studies are difficult to do and interpret in newborns. A muscle biopsy is usually required to make a specific diagnosis.

Molecular (deoxyribonucleic acid [DNA]) studies for certain diseases are now available, and if clinical suspicion is high, one may send these. A positive test avoids a muscle biopsy. Examples: Congenital myotonic dystrophy, spinal muscular atrophy, Duchenne's muscular dystrophy, etc., can be tested for using blood DNA analysis.

CASE CONTINUED

Labs: CBC: WNL. Electrolytes: WNL. CPK: 250 IU/mL.

**Muscle
biopsy:**   The left quadriceps is biopsied. Histopathology shows groups of atrophied (type 2) muscle fibers adjacent to hypertrophied type I fibers. This is evident on immunohistochemistry as well.

THOUGHT QUESTION

■ How does the work-up help further with the diagnosis?

        The work-up confirms a lower motor neuron process. A mild elevation of CPK suggests a primary muscle disorder, dystrophy, or anterior horn cell disease. A neuropathy is less likely. The muscle biopsy confirms the diagnosis of spinal muscular atrophy (SMA) type 1 (Werdnig-Hoffmann's disease).

QUESTIONS

34-1. Inheritance of spinal muscular atrophy is:
  A. Autosomal dominant
  B. Autosomal recessive
  C. X-linked dominant
  D. Multifactorial
  E. X-linked recessive

34-2. Etiology of peripheral hypotonia includes which of the following?
   A. Prader-Willi's syndrome
   B. Hypoxic-ischemic encephalopathy
   C. Down syndrome
   D. Cerebral dysgenesis
   E. Infant botulism

34-3. Which of the following is a sign of spasticity (as opposed to hypotonia)?
   A. Frog-leg position
   B. Head lag
   C. Scissoring of legs
   D. Scarf sign

34-4. The natural history of Werdnig-Hoffmann's disease is:
   A. Progressive weakness and death within 1 to 2 years of life
   B. Nonprogressive with static weakness
   C. Slowly progressive over many years
   D. Any of the above

ANSWERS

34-1. B. SMA is an autosomal recessive disease that affects the anterior horn cells. The classic and most extreme presentation is what is described in the case here, termed SMA type 1 or Werdnig-Hoffmann's disease, where an infant presents at birth or within the first 3 months with profound hypotonia, weakness, normal mentation, and absent deep tendon reflexes. Type 2 is the intermediate form of spinal muscular atrophy. It shares many features of Werdnig-Hoffmann's disease, but presents at a later age and has a slower course of progression. The disease can present even later in life, and the juvenile or chronic form (type 3) is called Kugelberg-Welander's disease. This form presents in late childhood or early adolescence, and has a less severe presentation and course.

34-2. E. Prader-Willi's syndrome, Down syndrome (trisomy 21) and hypoxic-ischemic encephalopathy are all examples of central (UMN) causes of hypotonia in a newborn. Infant botulism is a disorder of the neuromuscular junction caused by ingestion of spores of *Clostridium botulinum* and is characterized by muscle weakness and hypotonia, weak swallow, weak respiratory muscles, ophthalmoparesis, ptosis, and commonly constipation.

34-3. C. Frog-leg position, head lag, and the scarf sign are all signs of hypotonia rather than spasticity. Frog-leg position refers to the apparent posture of the legs when a hypotonic infant is placed supine. The legs lie flat against the bed, hips partially flexed and abducted, knees semiflexed, ankles partially dorsiflexed. Head lag refers to extension of the neck when the infant is pulled into a sitting position. Scarf sign is elicited by gently pulling the infant's arm across the midline. Normally the elbow does not cross the midline; in hypotonic infants it does so readily. Scissoring of legs refers to adduction at the hips resulting in a "scissored" or crossed posture of the legs is because of spasticity (hypertonia) in the lower extremities.

34-4. A. Werdnig-Hoffmann's disease is a progressive condition. Infants usually present within the first few months of life and get progressively weaker. Usually death results within the first 1 to 2 years of life from aspirations and respiratory failure.

 ADDITIONAL SUGGESTED READING

Chung BH, Wong VC, Ip P. Spinal muscular atrophy: survival pattern and functional status. Pediatrics 2004;114:e548.

Fox CK, Keet CA, Strober JB. Recent advances in infant botulism. Pediatr Neurol 2005;32:149.

Thompson JA, Filloux FM, Van Orman CB, et al. Infant botulism in the age of botulism immune globulin. Neurology 2005;64:2029.

VI

Patients Who Present with Trouble Walking, Leg Weakness, Numbness, or Pain

Paraparesis, Ataxia, and Incontinence

ID/CC: 48-year-old woman presents with progressive difficulty walking over the last 6 months and weakness in both legs.

HPI: About 6 months ago UI noticed that her right leg intermittently felt weak and occasionally would buckle underneath her. This slowly progressed to a sense of unsteadiness while walking. More recently she feels that her left leg has become weak as well and that her right leg occasionally stiffens up. On neurologic review of systems she also notes difficulty feeling the temperature of the water during her showers in her left leg and occasional band-like tightening sensations in right knee and ankle. Over the last week she has had three episodes of urinary incontinence.

PMHx: Gastroesophageal reflux disease

PSHx: Varicose vein removal

Meds: Tylenol (as needed) PRN

All: NKDA

SHx: She drinks two glasses of wine every day, does not smoke, lives with her boyfriend, works as a cashier, and has two adult children.

FHx: Maternal HTN, paternal unknown. Her brother underwent back surgery recently.

Neuro Hx: She diagnosed herself with migraine headaches that started 10 years ago. They occur approximately every 2 months and are relieved by rest and OTC pain relievers.

THOUGHT QUESTIONS

- How would you summarize the case thus far?
- Where could her lesion(s) localize? (at least three possibilities)
- What signs will you look for on examination to aid in localization?

Remember that for neurologic disorders, the timing of the onset of symptoms (acute, subacute, or chronic), the symmetry of symptoms, and whether the symptoms are intermittent (paroxysmal) or continuous are of key importance in generating a differential diagnosis. The case can be summarized as follows: 58-year-old woman with a subacute, progressive ataxia and asymmetric paraparesis accompanied by sensory changes in the left leg and urinary incontinence.

Given this information her lesion could localize to the cervical, thoracic, or lumbar spinal cord or to the bilateral medial frontal lobes. Multiple peripheral nerve involvement, as is seen in chronic inflammatory demyelinating polyneuropathy, is a much less likely possibility, because this process cannot explain urinary incontinence or the stiffening in her right leg that suggests spasticity (a UMN sign). A primary myopathic process again is not likely for the above reasons and because of the sensory involvement.

To aid in localization on examination, it is important to perform a thorough sensory evaluation with the patient undressed to look for a truncal sensory level and to assess superficial abdominal reflexes. Additionally, upper or lower motor neuron signs should be assessed as well as cognitive function. Lesions of the bilateral medial frontal lobes are usually accompanied by changes in cognitive function.

CASE CONTINUED

VS: Temp 98.6°F BP 110/70 HR 76 RR 16

PE: Gen: On skin examination, axillary freckles are noted.

Neuro: MSE: Patient is neatly groomed, mood is "okay" and affect is appropriate. MMSE is 30/30.

CN II–XII: Intact.

Motor: Normal bulk, tone, and strength in the bilateral upper extremities. Asymmetric weakness with increased tone in the legs as follows:

Reflexes: 3 and asymmetrical in the lower extremities, more pronounced on the right. 2 and equal in the upper extremities. Babinski signs present bilaterally.

Sensory: Severely diminished to pinprick and temperature sensation in the left leg and trunk up to the umbilicus. Light touch and vibration are slightly diminished in both legs up to the umbilicus.

Coordination: No tremor, nystagmus, or dysmetria is observed. Exam limited by lower extremity weakness.

Gait: Wide-based ataxia. Romberg sign is present.

 QUESTIONS

35-1. Which of the following is the most likely diagnosis?
A. Parasagittal meningioma
B. Spinal epidural neurofibroma
C. Bilateral frontal metastatic tumor
D. Cervical transverse myelitis
E. Syringomyelia

35-2. At what dermatome is her sensory level?
A. Th12
B. Th10
C. Th8
D. L2

35-3. Suppose her MRI scan reveals a large, asymmetric, intradural, extramedullary mass compressing the thoracic spinal cord. How should this patient be managed?
A. Emergent IV corticosteroids and radiotherapy (XRT)
B. Emergent surgery for removal of the mass
C. Whole-body scan and surgery for removal of the mass within the next week
D. IV high-dose corticosteroids

35-4. The patient undergoes surgery and the pathology shows wavy cells with elongated nuclei arranged in bundles with areas of palisading and whorling. What is her diagnosis?

- A. Neurofibromatosis type 1
- B. Neurofibromatosis type 2
- C. Meningioma
- D. Glioma

ANSWERS

35-1. B. In order to answer this question correctly the localization of the lesion needs to be clear. Given her history, the localization was narrowed to a spinal cord lesion or bilateral medial frontal lobe lesions. Her examination clearly points to a spinal cord lesion rather than a cerebral process. She has a discrete, truncal sensory level, preserved upper extremity strength and reflexes, and intact cognition. Bilateral medial frontal lobe lesions will not give you sensory changes. Her examination and history tell you that she has a subacute progressive myelopathy, which can be because of either an intramedullary or extramedullary (compressive) spinal cord lesion. The asymmetry of the onset of symptoms (right leg spastic weakness); early, asymmetric involvement of the spinothalamic tract (contralateral pain and temperature loss) and band-like pains around the right knee and ankle are classic findings of an extramedullary, compressive process. Symptoms of intramedullary spinal cord lesions, such as syringomyelia and ependymomas, usually begin with symmetric band-like painful sensations and loss of pain and temperature sensation because of involvement of the decussation of the spinothalamic tracts. Weakness is also usually symmetric, and bladder function is usually spared. Transverse myelitis, usually because of demyelinating disease or an infectious/postinfectious process, can present with either type of symptoms. Although it is an intrinsic spinal cord process, it does not always involve the entire level and can be more centrally or asymmetrically located.

35-2. B. The umbilicus is typically located in the 10th thoracic dermatome. Remember that this means the spinal cord lesion itself can localize to two levels above and below the sensory level (in this case Th8–Th12) because the spinothalamic tracts ascend ipsilaterally for a short course before decussating. This is often referred to as a "false localizing sign."

35-3. B. This patient should go to emergent surgery for removal of the mass because she has early bladder involvement. Once bladder impairment exceeds 2 weeks it is unlikely that it can be regained even if the mass is removed. The longer one waits to remove the mass the less likely it is she will be able to regain her bladder function.

35-4. A. This patient has neurofibromatosis type 1 (von Recklinghausen neurofibromatosis or general NF). To meet the criteria for this diagnosis in adults two of the following clinical features must be present: (1) six or more café-au-lait spots over 15 mm; (2) axillary or inguinal freckles; (3) optic nerve or chiasmatic glioma; (4) two or more Lisch iris nodules; (5) thinning of long-bone cortex; (6) dysplasia of the sphenoid; (7) one plexiform neurofibroma or two neurofibromas of any type; or (8) a first-degree relative with NF 1. In neurofibromatosis type 2, the hallmarks are schwannomas involving the cranial or spinal roots leading to progressive compression and bilateral or, less commonly, unilateral acoustic neuromas. It is associated with cutaneous neurofibromas, meningiomas, glioma, and café-au-lait spots but not axillary freckles. The characteristic pathologic findings in meningiomas are round, calcified psammoma bodies. Neurofibromas are the most common intradural, extramedullary lesions found in the thoracic spinal cord in adults, with meningiomas being the second most common. Much more rare are metastases. NF 1 is the most common genetic disorder affecting the nervous system, with an estimated prevalence of 1 in 3,000 people. It is usually autosomal dominant and is located on chromosome 17q. She should undergo a brain MRI not only to look for occult optic gliomas but also because in 5% to 10% of people NF 1 is associated with intracranial meningiomas and schwannomas. Her history of headaches is suspicious of a possible intracranial lesion. Neurofibromas of the spinal cord are often multiple and therefore she should have her remaining spinal cord imaged as well.

 ADDITIONAL SUGGESTED READING

Custer BS, Koepsell TD, Mueller BA. The association between breast carcinoma and meningioma in women. Cancer 2002;94:1626.
Whittle IR, Smith C, Navoo P, et al. Meningiomas. Lancet 2004;363:1535.

Leg Pain and Urinary Incontinence

ID/CC: 49-year-old woman who presents with sciatic pain, constipation, and urinary incontinence

HPI: Approximately 1 month ago ME developed sciatic pain radiating down into her buttock and vaginal area. Additionally, she has the concomitant complaints of constipation and diminished urine stream and control.

PMHx: None

PSHx: Tonsillectomy

Meds: None

All: NKDA

Habits: Smoked half a pack of cigarettes per day for 15 years, no alcohol, no IVDA, or recreational drugs

VS: BP 132/74 HR 87 RR 12

PE/Neuro: No deficits in strength or sensation or reflexes. There is marked rectal laxity.

THOUGHT QUESTIONS

- What is the differential diagnosis?
- What additional studies would you obtain?

The patient's symptoms are concerning for a spinal cord lesion that is causing canal compromise and affecting associated nerve roots. The differential diagnosis includes ependymoma, astrocytoma, dermoid and epidermoid, lipoma, metastases, and infection. To better clarify the diagnosis, a MRI of the lumbosacral spine is the preferred study. An MRI is a more sensitive study for the evaluation of the dura, cord, and associated soft tissues and ligaments. Should it not be possible to obtain an MRI, a CT scan with and without contrast may also be of assistance.

CASE CONTINUED

Her primary care physician ordered an MRI of the lumbosacral spine and performed a lumbar puncture before referring the patient for further treatment (Fig. 36-1).

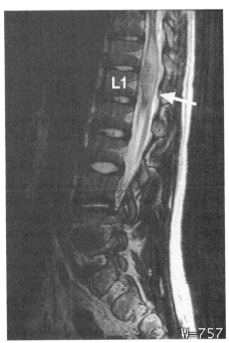

FIGURE 36-1
MRI of the lumbosacral spine: The conus medullaris is enlarged. Following contrast there is a 1-cm intramedullary lesion at the level of L1 extending from the conus into the filum. It is strongly ring enhancing. (*Image provided by the Departments of Neuroradiology and Neurosurgery, Stanford University, Stanford, California.*)

MRI of the lumbosacral spine: The conus medullaris is enlarged. Following contrast there is a 1 cm intramedullary lesion at the level of L1 extending from the conus into the filum. It is strongly ring enhancing.

Lumbar puncture: CSF—protein is elevated at 192, glucose and leukocytes are WNL.

THOUGHT QUESTIONS

■ What is the patient's differential diagnosis now that we have CSF and MRI findings?

■ Which of the potential diagnosis is most consistent with the CSF findings?

The differential diagnosis as noted above includes ependymoma, astrocytoma, dermoid and epidermoid, lipoma, metastases, and infection.

The radiographic images are inconsistent with a lipoma. In addition, although small lipomas may be found in the film, the majority are located in the cervical and thoracic spine. The signal characteristics on MRI are also inconsistent with either dermoid or epidermoid.

Although metastases to the spine may be intramedullary, the vast majority are extradural and the preferred location is the thoracic spine.

The CSF findings are inconsistent with an infectious etiology.

Thus the two most likely diagnoses are astrocytoma and ependymoma. Ependymomas are the most common primary spinal cord tumor, followed by astrocytomas. There is no specific aspect of the history or radiographic images that is reliable in differentiating the two tumors.

The findings are consistent with an intramedullary spinal cord tumor. Elevated protein is the most common abnormality identified. Glucose is also usually normal.

CASE CONTINUED

An MRI of the head is also obtained and there is no evidence of an intracerebral lesion. All treatment options were reviewed and the decision is made to undergo a biopsy of the lesion. This is performed without complication. The pathology identifies a myxopapillary ependymoma.

QUESTIONS

36-1. What is the most common location of myxopapillary ependymomas?
   A. Thoracic spine
   B. Cervical spine
   C. Filum terminale
   D. Medulla

36-2. Which of the following neurocutaneous syndromes is associated with spinal ependymomas?
   A. Neurofibromatosis type 2 (NF 2)
   B. Sturge-Weber
   C. Von Hippel-Lindau's disease
   D. None of the above

36-3. Which of the following is the most common presentation of myxopapillary ependymomas?
   A. Sphincter disturbance
   B. Leg weakness
   C. Pain
   D. None of the above

36-4. Which of the following statements is consistent with myxopapillary ependymomas?
   A. Myxopapillary ependymomas may grow to be extremely large.
   B. Myxopapillary ependymomas never erode bone.
   C. CSF dissemination commonly occurs with myxopapillary ependymomas.
   D. None of the above

 ANSWERS

36-1. C. Ependymomas may occur anywhere along the neuraxis. In the spine the cervical cord is the most common site for intramedullary ependymomas. The typical location for myxopapillary ependymomas is the filum terminale.

36-2. A. Myxopapillary ependymomas are associated with neurofibromatosis type 2. NF 2 and Sturge-Weber are both neurocutaneous disorders. Sturge-Weber is classically associated with a facial port wine nevus and cortical cerebral atrophy. Von Hippel-Lindau's disease is characterized by the presence of hemangioblastomas, renal cell carcinomas, retinal angiomas, and polycythemia.

36-3. C. Patients with spinal ependymomas present with a variety of clinical symptoms, including leg weakness and sphincter disturbance. Back pain is the most common presenting symptom.

36-4. A. Myxopapillary ependymomas, although slow growing, may grow to extremely large sizes and erode bone. It is a rare occurrence that myxopapillary ependymomas disseminate via the CSF.

 ADDITIONAL SUGGESTED READING

Kleihues P, Burger PC, Collins VP, et al. Glioblastoma. In: Kleihues P, Cavenee WK, eds. Pathology of the Nervous System: World Health Organization Classification of Tumors. Lyon, France: IARC (International Agency for Research on Cancer), 2000:29.

Chronic Progressive Difficulty Walking

ID/CC: 68-year-old woman presents with increasing difficulty walking over the last 20 years.

HPI: MW first noticed difficulty climbing ladders about 20 years ago. Around the same time she also noticed occasional difficulty letting go of frying pans while she was preparing dinner. She then developed difficulty climbing stairs and more recently rising out of a chair. Her symptoms progressed very slowly, without any dramatic fluctuations or periods of decline. For the last year MW has required a walker for ambulation. She has fallen multiple times. On neurologic review of systems she states she has "always been clumsy," frequently tripping and dropping things since her teen years. She also occasionally has minor difficulty swallowing and chewing. She denies any numbness, tingling, or pain. No double vision, change in voice or handwriting. No bowel, bladder, or sexual dysfunction. No history of trauma.

PM/SHx: Hypothyroidism

Meds: Synthroid

All: NKDA

SHx: Married, no children, desired but only able to conceive one child that was stillborn at term. Housewife. Drinks two glasses of wine a night. Does not smoke.

FHx: Unknown. Patient is adopted.

VS: Temp 98.6°F BP 130/70 HR 88

PE: Gen: Thin, well-groomed woman. No carotid bruits. No lymphadenopathy.

Lungs: CTA. COR: RRR no murmurs

Abdomen: Soft, NT, nondistended, no organomegaly, no bruits.

Extremities: No erythema, edema, or tenderness

Skin: No rashes

Neuro: CN II–X, XII: intact. Symmetrical sternocleidomastoid weakness. Fundi not visualized.

Motor: Tone is normal to slightly diminished. Atrophy of the masseter, temporalis, and sternocleidomastoid muscles. Strength as follows (out of 5); neck flexion and extension, 4; shoulder abduction, external and internal rotation, 5; shoulder adduction, 4; triceps, 5; biceps, 4; wrist flexors, 4; extensors, 5; finger flexors and extensors, 4; hip flexors, 3; extensors, 4; knee extension and flexion, 4; plantar flexion, 4; dorsiflexion, 3. Difficulty rising out of a chair. Percussion of the thenar eminence reveals no myotonia. No fasciculations are present.

Reflexes: 2+ biceps, triceps, brachioradialis, and patella; 1+ at the ankles. Babinski signs absent bilaterally.

Sensory: Intact to light touch, pinprick, temperature, and vibration in all four extremities

Coordination: No tremor, nystagmus, or dysmetria is present.

Gait: Ambulates with a walker. Stance is normal. Unable to walk on heels. Toe walking intact. High steppage, shuffling gait.

THOUGHT QUESTIONS

- Summarize the case thus far.
- Discuss a general approach for evaluating patients with weakness in the absence of marked upper or lower motor neuron signs.
- What is myotonia?

This is an elderly woman with chronic weakness affecting the distal and proximal limb girdle muscles, neck flexors, masseter, and temporalis with relatively preserved muscle tone and reflexes. The proximal weakness in her legs began during middle age. She has hypothyroidism, probably infertility, and one full-term stillbirth.

No sensory or cerebellar abnormalities are present. While she has complained of symptoms consistent with myotonia in her hands in the past, she does not have any in her thenar eminence on exam. The chronic, slowly progressive course of her illness is highly suggestive of a hereditary illness.

A useful approach to evaluating patients with weakness in the absence of marked upper or motor neuron signs as in this patient follows:

1. First, decide whether the weakness is constant or fluctuating. Fluctuating weakness is caused by neuromuscular junction disorders (myasthenia gravis or Lambert-Eaton's syndrome), periodic paralysis, and metabolic myopathies.
2. If the weakness is constant, determine whether it is chronic constant weakness or acquired chronic weakness. The differential diagnosis for chronic acquired weakness includes polymyositis, dermatomyositis, inclusion body myositis, multifocal motor neuropathy, and ALS. ALS over time will become easy to distinguish from other disorders because obvious upper and lower motor neuron signs will develop.
3. If the weakness has been chronic (often lifelong) and constant then determine whether it is progressive or static (nonprogressive). Static lifelong (chronic) weakness is most likely because of a congenital myopathy or congenital dystrophy.
4. For lifelong progressive weakness with or without lower motor neuron signs important clues to the etiology are the presence of:
   a. Ocular weakness (ocular dystrophy, oculopharyngeal dystrophy and Kearns-Sayers' syndrome)
   b. Facial weakness (myotonic dystrophy and facioscapulohumeral dystrophy)
   c. Upper extremity weakness predominating (Emery-Dreifuss dystrophy and hereditary distal myopathy)

Lower extremity weakness predominating (Becker and Duchenne muscular dystrophy, spinal muscular atrophy, and limb girdle dystrophy). Myotonia is the slowed relaxation of muscle contraction following percussion or voluntary contraction because of hyperexcitability of the muscle membrane. Clinically, it usually involves the hands and tongue and patients may complain of difficulty releasing objects after voluntarily grasping them and difficulty chewing. Other complaints that can arise because of myotonia are difficulty climbing ladders or stairs quickly despite lack of weakness on direct muscle group testing and inability to open the mouth while eating. Most patients do not complain of myotonia and must be questioned specifically to elicit this history.

CASE CONTINUED

Serum CK—200 mU/mL (upper limit of normal is 145); EMG/NCV show diffuse small, polyphasic motor unit action potentials, fibrillations, and increased insertional activity with high-frequency bursts of muscle action potentials in the deltoid muscles. Nerve conduction amplitudes and velocities are normal. No conduction blocks are present.

 QUESTIONS

37-1. What is the most likely diagnosis?
- A. Myotonia congenita
- B. Myotonic dystrophy
- C. Limb girdle dystrophy
- D. Manifest carrier of DMD

37-2. Which of the following abnormalities is associated with her illness?
- A. Cataracts
- B. Mental retardation
- C. Infertility
- D. All of the above

37-3. This disorder is inherited in which manner?
- A. Autosomal dominant mutation
- B. Autosomal recessive mutation
- C. X-linked triplicate repeat expansion
- D. Autosomal dominant triplicate repeat expansion

37-4. Which of the following is true regarding her disease?
- A. The disease is more severe when inherited from the father.
- B. There is an increased risk of general anesthetic complications.
- C. Proximal muscles are more commonly involved than distal muscles.
- D. Within a family the phenotype usually remains stable.

 ANSWERS

37-1. B. This patient most likely has myotonic dystrophy (MD). MD is the most common hereditary myopathy seen in adults and occurs in 1:8,000 live births. Distinguishing characteristics from other hereditary muscular dystrophies presenting in adulthood are the prominent involvement of facial muscles and neck muscles and early involvement of distal limb muscles. The myotonia in the hands often disappears as the disease progresses although it is often still evident in other muscle groups such as the deltoids. Myotonia congenita is a nonprogressive channelopathy whose main clinical feature is disabling myotonia, resulting in stiffness with most voluntary movements, not weakness.

37-2. D. MD involves other organs as well. Cataracts and cardiac involvement are very common, as are endocrine abnormalities of the testes, pancreas, hypothalamus and thyroid; insulin resistance; and frequent spontaneous miscarriages. Cardiac arrhythmias and an unusual dilated cardiomyopathy may account for the high risk of sudden death in patients with MD. Intellectual function in people with MD can range from normal IQ to severe mental retardation. In the case of severe mental retardation, the diagnosis of MD can be missed.

37-3. D, **37-4.** B. MD is inherited in an autosomal dominant fashion and is caused by a cervicothoracic ganglion (CTG) triplicate repeat expansion in the gene encoding for a serine threonine kinase on chromosome 19q. Normal individuals have 5 to 30 CTG repeats in this region while patients with MD have hundreds to thousands. Like other triplicate repeat diseases (including Huntington's disease, Friedreich ataxia, and Fragile X syndrome) the phenomenon of genetic anticipation is often seen. This means that as the repeat is passed down it usually undergoes expansion and causes a more severe phenotype in the offsprings of affected individuals. Patients with MD are at increased risk of developing cardiac arrhythmias and malignant hyperthermia following general anesthesia.

 ADDITIONAL SUGGESTED READING

Darras BT, Friedman NR. Metabolic myopathies: a clinical approach; part I. Pediatr Neurol 2000;22:87.

Duyff RF, Van den BJ, Laman DM, et al. Neuromuscular findings in thyroid dysfunction: a prospective clinical and electrodiagnostic study. J Neurol Neurosurg Psychiatry 2000;68:750.

Sieb JP, Gillessen T. Iatrogenic and toxic myopathies. Muscle Nerve 2003;27:142.

Child Late in Walking

ID/CC: 16-month-old child, not walking as yet.

HPI: NC is a 16-month-old female who was evaluated for not walking.

Pregnancy was notable for hyperemesis in the first trimester, mild HTN at 37 weeks. Labor was induced for HTN at 38 weeks. The baby was born vaginally with Apgar scores of 8 at 1 minute and 9 at 5 minutes. No neonatal complications. The baby was discharged home with her mother on day two of life.

She began smiling at 6 to 7 weeks of age. By 4 months of age, her neck was steady and did not wobble as much when she was lifted. She began batting at her mobile over the crib at 4 months and cooing at things and in response to mom or dad around the same time. By 7 months of age, she was sitting supported, and by 9 months of age was sitting unsupported and scooting forward on her abdomen. She would pull herself to stand by 11 months of age, but had not started walking at the time of presentation.

PMHx: Otitis media at 7 months of age

Meds: None

All: None

FHx: Noncontributory

SHx: Only child of parents. Both parents are employed in the software industry.

PE: Gen: normal

Neuro: Normal

VS: WNL. Weight 11 kg (50th percentile), length: OFC 45.5 cm (10th–25th percentile)

THOUGHT QUESTION

■ What areas of development will you assess?

Commonly assessed areas of development are gross motor, fine motor, language, and social/cognitive areas.

Gross motor: Here, motor skills such as rolling over, sitting, crawling, etc. are assessed. A normal baby shows stable head control at 4 months of age, rolls over by 5 months, sits unassisted by 6 to 7 months. Many babies will scoot forward on their abdomen, i.e., "commando crawl" by this age. Crawling begins by 8 to 9 months. In the next few months, infants begin to pull to a standing position, stand unassisted, and then gradually begin walking by 12 to 15 months.

Fine motor: Skills assessed include grasping toys by 3 to 4 months of age, bringing hands together by 4 to 5 months, and transferring objects from one hand to the other. A crude "raking" grasp appears by 7 months, and a more refined pincer grasp by 9 to 10 months. By 1 year of age, infants can finger feed and put objects in a cup.

Language: Cooing and gurgling begins at 2 to 3 months. Single-syllable words appear by 6 months. By 9 months, words like "dada and mama" appear. Closer to 12 months, "dada" and "mama" begin to be used specifically. On average, a 12-month-old will have at least one word in his or her vocabulary.

Social/cognitive: Social smile appears at 6 weeks of age. By 3 to 4 months babies regard their own hands, and later their feet.

This child shows steady developmental progress in all four areas. Her development in fine motor, cognitive, and language areas is normal. Her walking, although "late" by strict criteria, is really the only milestone that is "delayed." In the face of a normal neurologic examination a single apparently delayed milestone does not warrant a big diagnostic work-up. Close follow-up is however necessary.

CASE CONTINUED

The child is asked to follow up after 6 months. At her follow-up visit she is doing the following:

Motor: Walking without support, crawling up and down stairs

Fine motor: Feeds herself using a cup and fingers. "Makes a mess" with a spoon, but shows interest in using one. Builds a tower of four cubes.

Language: Vocabulary of 30 words. Not putting two words together yet.

**Social/
Cognitive:**   Helps with dressing herself. She likes playing with her dolls, especially feeding them and putting them to bed.

Examination is entirely normal.

Conclusion: This is a developmentally normal 22-month-old child.

No further work-up is necessary.

     QUESTIONS

38-1. Which of the following reflexes appears after the neonatal period and persists throughout adult life?
   A. Moro reflex
   B. Parachute reflex
   C. Stepping and placing reflexes
   D. Landau reflex

38-2. Head circumference in an 8-month-old child with a head circumference of 34 cm at birth should measure approximately:
   A. 38 cm
   B. 40 cm
   C. 44 cm
   D. 47 cm
   E. 49 cm

38-3. Which of the following should prompt concern if seen on developmental assessment of a 9-month-old child?
   A. Object permanence
   B. Couple of monosyllable words like "mama"
   C. Parachute reflex
   D. Raking grasp

38-4. By 2 years a child's language development should have the following feature:
   A. 15-word vocabulary
   B. Puts two words together
   C. Speaks in short phrases
   D. Speech easily understood by all

ANSWERS

38-1. B. Neonates have a number of primitive reflexes that are lost as the infant grows and acquires new developmental skills. The moro reflex is a reaction to a startle stimulus (e.g., loud noise, sudden touch, sudden lowering of the entire body) in which the infant's arms and legs abduct and the hands open. In the stepping or placing reflex, when the dorsal (back) side of the hand or foot is placed on the edge of a surface, such as a table, the infant will lift the extremity and place it on the flat surface The Landau reflex is elicited by placing the child in a horizontal, prone suspension. The child will extend his neck, head, and arms. Lower extremities are flexed. Moro reflex, stepping and placing reflexes and Landau's reflex are all primitive reflexes seen in normal, full-term neonates. These disappear by 3 months of age. The parachute reflex occurs when the patient is lowered toward a surface in the prone position; the normal response is to extend the arms and hands to cushion the fall. The parachute reflex appears at around 9 months of age and persists lifelong.

38-2. C. The average rate of head circumference increase in the first year of life for a term infant is 2 cm per month for the first 3 months, 1 cm per month for the next 3 months, and 0.5 cm per months for the next 6 months. Thus an infant with a head circumference of 34 cm at birth should add about 10 cm by 8 months of age. Therefore the infant's head circumference should measure approximately 44 cm.

38-3. D. At 9 months, an infant shows interest in objects that are taken away from his/her field of vision and will seek them when this is done. This refers to object permanence. The parachute reflex appears at this age and persists for life. A few monosyllable words are common by this age. The infant should have a pincer grasp by 9 months of age, not a raking grasp.

38-4. B. By 2 years, a child should have a vocabulary of 50 words, be able to put 2 words together, and his/her speech should be understood 50% of the time.

ADDITIONAL SUGGESTED READING

Swaiman KF. Pediatric Neurology: Principles and Practice, 2nd ed. St. Louis: Mosby, 1989:205.

Child Clumsy in Walking

 ID/CC: 5-year-old boy with clumsy walking.

HPI: CK, a 5-year-old boy presents with clumsy walking. He was first noted to have trouble walking at 2 years of age. He was slower to walk than his peers, not walking independently until 19 months of age. His walking was always wide-based and steps uncertain. He had trouble learning to climb stairs, and began doing so at age 3 and a half years. Now, at 5 years of age he is still slow to climb stairs, and has trouble running. He has no difficulty using utensils to eat, putting on shirt buttons, and his speech is age appropriate. He is scheduled to begin kindergarten in the fall.

PMHx: Seasonal allergies

Meds: Claritin

All: NKDA

FHx: Noncontributory

SHx: Has an older sister who is normal

PE: Gen: normal

Neuro: Mental status: Alert, fluent and age appropriate speech. Cranial nerve examination: normal. Normal funduscopic examination.

Motor: Muscle tone mildly low

Strength: 4/5 in deltoids, shoulder flexion, and extension. Biceps, triceps, and more distal arm and hand muscles 5/5. Hip flexors and extensors 4/5, rest of lower extremity muscles 5/5. He has a positive Gower sign.

Reflexes: 1+ bilaterally symmetric. Plantar flexor. Normal sensory examination, coordination. His lower extremity muscles seem rather well-developed for a child who is mildly weak on examination; in fact his calf muscles look rather big.

VS: Normal

THOUGHT QUESTIONS

- What is your differential diagnosis?
- What lab tests will be helpful making a diagnosis?
- What is Gower sign?

Key points in this case are delayed motor development with normal speech and fine motor development, and seemingly normal cognition. The normal intellect and lack of upper motor neuron signs on examination make this unlikely to be a central UMN process.

The patient's examination is notable for proximal motor weakness, low muscle tone, and diminished reflexes. These findings suggest a lower motor neuron lesion. Proximal muscle weakness is characteristic of a myopathy, versus distal weakness, which is suggestive of a neuropathy. The presence of reflexes makes anterior horn cell disease unlikely. The lack of fatigable muscle weakness or ocular muscle involvement makes neuromuscular disease less likely.

Given this background, tests that help to delineate these conditions further include muscle enzyme studies, EMG/NCV studies, and, if needed, a nerve/muscle biopsy.

When asked to stand up from a supine position, the patient will first turn to one side, then use his hands to support himself as he gets up. As he gets into a standing position, he will place his hands on his thighs, then waist to support himself. This manner in which the patient rises from supine to standing position indicates weakness of the hip girdle. It was described by Gower and is hence termed "Gower sign."

CASE CONTINUED

Labs: CBC: WNL. Electrolytes: WNL. AST: 250. CPK: 10,400 IU/mL. Muscle biopsy: Shows regions of degenerating muscle fibers and regions of regenerating fibers, fatty infiltration in the muscle.

THOUGHT QUESTION

- How do these labs help with the differential diagnosis further?

The laboratory data indicates that this is a primary muscle disorder. Elevations in muscle enzymes are seen in myopathies, where creatine phosphokinase (CPK) elevation is commonly several hundred or a few thousand IU/mL. Smaller elevations can be seen in anterior horn cell disease and neuropathic conditions.

The marked elevation of CPK along with calf muscle hypertrophy is virtually diagnostic of a muscular dystrophy. The muscle biopsy confirms the dystrophy. This presentation is characteristic for DMD.

DMD is a genetically inherited muscular dystrophy. Clinical features include proximal weakness, more prominent in the legs than in the arms. Reflexes are preserved early in the course of the disease. The dystrophic process causes pseudohypertrophy of calf muscles. Other muscles affected include deltoid and quadriceps and sometimes tongue muscles. Serum CPK is elevated into the thousands early in the course of the disease. Later in the course, CPK levels fall, but do not become normal.

QUESTIONS

39-1. Inheritance of DMD is:
- A. Autosomal dominant
- B. Autosomal recessive
- C. X-linked recessive
- D. Multifactorial

39-2. Becker muscular dystrophy presents at what age?
- A. Infancy
- B. 3 to 5 years
- C. 12 to 14 years
- D. 20 to 25 years

39-3. Work-up for DMD should also include the following:
A. ECG
B. MRI brain
C. Dilated eye examination
D. Renal ultrasound

39-4. Natural history of DMD includes:
A. Scoliosis
B. Progressive weakness
C. Cardiomyopathy and respiratory compromise
D. All of the above

ANSWERS

39-1. C. DMD is X-linked recessive in its inheritance. This means that boys are affected, while mothers are carriers. Mothers of affected boys may show a modest increase in serum CPK levels, and may be asymptomatic. The gene associated with DMD is located on the long arm of chromosome 21, resulting in reduced or abnormal production of dystrophin.

39-2. C. Becker muscular dystrophy presents in pre- or early adolescence. In its clinical symptomatology it is similar to DMD. Muscle histology is also the same. This type of muscular dystrophy has a relatively more indolent course, with life expectancy in the 30s to 40s. Recently milder expressions of DMD/Becker muscular dystrophy have been identified, with the same biochemical and genetic defects. The entire spectrum is termed "dystrophinopathies."

39-3. A. In DMD, the degenerative process is not limited to skeletal muscles, although they are most prominently affected. Cardiac muscle dysfunction also occurs in the course of the disease. A baseline cardiac evaluation is usually recommended in these patients. Some degree of intellectual impairment may also be present, but an MRI scan of the brain is not mandatory in the work-up. There are other, rare forms of muscular dystrophy where intellectual impairment, seizures, and visual impairment are present and in these MRI scan of the brain and/or eye examinations are performed.

39-4. D. DMD is a chronic progressive disease. Progressive weakness of skeletal muscles occurs over time, making walking more difficult, and at some point these children get confined to a wheelchair. Spine scoliosis also occurs in the course of the disease, and tends to progress once the child is in a wheelchair. Cardiomyopathy results over time from cardiac muscle involvement. Skeletal muscle weakness, scoliosis, and cardiomyopathy all contribute to respiratory compromise over time.

 ADDITIONAL SUGGESTED READING

Emery AE. The muscular dystrophies. Lancet 2002;359:687.
Moxley RT 3rd, Ashwal S, Pandya S, et al. Practice parameter: corticosteroid treatment of Duchenne dystrophy: report of the Quality Standards Subcommittee of the American Academy of Neurology and the Practice Committee of the Child Neurology Society. Neurology 2005;64:13.

Low Back Pain

ID/CC: 82-year-old woman who presents with 2-month history of pain in her lower back

HPI: IC complains that after walking two to three blocks she develops significant discomfort in her lower back. She describes both pain and tingling that radiate down the lateral aspect of both thighs and then to the medial aspect of her legs. She notes that standing for long periods also exacerbates these symptoms. Her symptoms are improved when she stops walking and sits or reclines for at least 30 minutes. The patient also reports relief when she flexes at the waist in a stooped posture.

PMHx: HTN, Afib

PSHx: None

Meds: Hyzaar

All: NKDA

SHx: The patient lives with her son and his family. She walks daily and swims twice weekly.

Habits: No tobacco, no alcohol, no IVDA or recreational drugs

THOUGHT QUESTIONS

- Based on this history, what is the differential diagnosis?
- What areas of the neurologic and PE would you now focus on to better clarify your differential?

The patient presents with a history of pain and abnormal sensations in her lower back, thighs, and legs. To assess abnormalities of sensation, specific aspects of the history are important. A clear description of these sensory symptoms is essential. The described tingling and numbness are among the abnormal sensations encompassed by the term paresthesias. Others include the abnormal sensation of burning and/or pins and needles. It is also important to note the onset, duration, and progression of symptoms, their exacerbating and alleviating factors, and any associated complaints. Further, the specific location and distribution of the symptoms will help in localizing the origin of the complaint. The past medical and surgical histories are also important. Notable in this patient's history is the absence of systemic malignancy, trauma, and peripheral vascular disease. The symptoms given are suggestive of several conditions including lumbar spinal stenosis, vascular insufficiency, disc herniation, intraspinal tumor, and arachnoiditis.

CASE CONTINUED

VS: Temp 98.8°F BP 134/84 HR 80 RR 12

PE/Neuro: The patient's legs have normal pallor both at rest and with elevation. The peripheral pulses are strong bilaterally. The patient has normal strength in all motor groups of the lower extremities. There is decreased sensation in the L3–L4 dermatomal distribution. The patellar reflexes are diminished bilaterally. Straight leg raising test (Lasègue's sign) and reverse straight leg raising are negative bilaterally.

THOUGHT QUESTIONS

- What clinical syndrome is most consistent with the given history and PE?
- What radiographic studies would be helpful in establishing a diagnosis?

The patient's history is consistent with claudication. Claudication is defined as intermittent pain ± weakness, ± radicular sensory abnormalities. The symptoms usually present with activity and are relieved by rest. Differentiating between neurogenic and vascular claudication is essential. Several aspects of the H&P are consistent with neurogenic claudication. Unlike vascular claudication, the distribution of pain and sensory loss is dermatomal, and the symptoms are relieved with rest over a period of time. Other significant findings are the absence of pallor, the presence of peripheral pulses, and normal temperature of the feet, all of which are inconsistent with vascular claudication.

The lumbosacral spine radiographs, CT, and MRI scans will help in identifying the etiology of the patient's symptoms. The radiographs and CT scan will focus on the bony anatomy of the lumbosacral spine. The CT scan will best outline bony and ligamentous hypertrophy. The MRI is best at assessing the associated soft tissue and in identifying the presence/absence of associated malignancy or mass lesion. The patient has a pacemaker. This is a contraindication for obtaining an MRI. Other relative contraindications include the presence of shrapnel, ferromagnetic implants, and weight in excess of 300 pounds, as some machines have weight limits. Claustrophobia, once a relative contraindication, may be addressed with sedatives or the use of an open scanner (also used for obese patients). In this case, a CT scan is advised.

 CASE CONTINUED

The lumbosacral spine radiograph demonstrates a congenitally narrowed spinal canal further narrowed by bony hypertrophy. The CT scan further demonstrates a decreased AP diameter of the spinal canal secondary to a combination of facet hypertrophy and hypertrophy of the ligamentum flavum (Fig. 40-1).

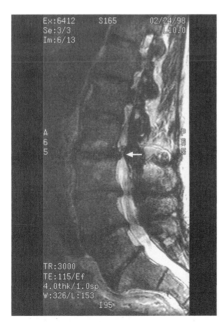

FIGURE **40-1**
The lumbosacral spine MRI demonstrates a congenitally narrowed spinal canal further narrowed by bony hypertrophy. The MRI scan further demonstrates a decreased AP diameter of the spinal canal secondary to a combination of facet hypertrophy and hypertrophy of the ligamentum flavum. (*Image provided by the Departments of Neuroradiology and Neurosurgery, University of California, San Francisco.*)

Conservative measures were attempted including NSAIDs and physical therapy. After an 8-week trial, the patient is without improvement. She returns once again to the clinic. On further discussion, the decision is made to undergo surgical decompression. A lumbar laminectomy is performed. On follow-up the patient reports absence of pain and improvement in paresthesias. She has resumed her daily walking regimen.

 QUESTIONS

40-1. Which of the following is most likely to lead to symptomatic lumbar stenosis?
- A. A congenital abnormality
- B. Diabetes
- C. Short-term steroid use
- D. History of HTN

40-2. Which of the following is consistent with a diagnosis of neurogenic claudication?
- A. Stocking distribution of sensory loss
- B. Diminished peripheral pulses
- C. Abnormal pallor of the feet
- D. Anthropoid posture

40-3. Which of the following conditions is associated with lumbar stenosis?
- A. Achondroplasia
- B. HTN
- C. Asthma
- D. Congestive heart failure

40-4. What is the gold standard in the management of patients with lumbar stenosis?
- A. Surgical decompression
- B. NSAIDs
- C. Steroids
- D. None of the above

 ANSWERS

40-1. A. Lumbar spinal stenosis may result from any of a number of conditions that critically narrow the AP diameter of the spinal canal. Although the canal may be congenitally narrowed or narrowed from congenital causes such as achondroplasia, other acquired conditions may result in stenosis. These causes include spondylolisthesis, arachnoiditis, disc herniation, and acromegaly. Additionally, prolonged steroid use has been associated with a condition known as epidural lipomatosis, that may result in narrowing of the spinal canal and symptoms associated with spinal stenosis. Diabetes, short-term steroid use, and HTN are not known to lead to spinal stenosis.

40-2. D. The presence of diminished peripheral pulses, abnormal pallor of the feet, and stocking distribution of sensory loss are all consistent with vascular claudication. Anthropoid posture is most consistent with neurogenic claudication. (Also see discussion above under thought questions.)

40-3. A. Achondroplasia is a congenital disorder associated with lumbar spinal stenosis. It is an autosomal dominant disorder caused by a mutation in the gene for fibroblast growth factor (FGF) receptor 3, leading to reduction in the proliferation of chondrocytes in the growth plate. It manifests clinically as dwarfism, but the abnormal development of vertebrae may lead to spinal stenosis. HTN, asthma, and congestive heart failure are not associated with lumbar spinal stenosis.

40-4. D. In the management of lumbar stenosis treatment is guided by the specifics of the history, physical, and neurologic examinations, and radiographic findings. There is no gold standard for care. A significant percentage of patients with lumbar stenosis will recover with conservative management. Indications for surgical intervention include, but are not limited to, failure of conservative measures to improve the patients' symptoms, or progressive neurologic deficit while being managed conservatively.

 ADDITIONAL SUGGESTED READING

Beattie PF, Meyers SP, Stratford P, et al. Associations between patient report of symptoms and anatomic impairment visible on lumbar magnetic resonance imaging. Spine 2000;25:819.

Hammerberg KW. New concepts on the pathogenesis and classification of spondylolisthesis. Spine 2005;30:S4.

Right Ankle Weakness

ID/CC: 26-year-old woman presents with acute onset of right ankle weakness.

HPI: KS was sitting in a conference yesterday with her legs crossed for about an hour. After the conference ended she was unable to stand up because of severe weakness in her right ankle. She is 4 months postpartum following a prolonged second stage of labor resulting in a forceps delivery. She has recently lost all 40 pounds that she gained during pregnancy. On neurologic review of systems, she denies any numbness, tingling, or pain in her legs; no change in bowel, bladder, or sexual function; no weakness in her arms or left leg. No muscle cramping. She has had similar episodes in the past but the weakness was never as severe and usually resolved within 10 minutes.

PMHx: None

PSHx: None

Meds: None

All: NKDA

SHx: Married, works full-time, has one healthy 4-month-old son. Does not drink or smoke. No history of IVDA.

FHx: No family history of neurologic illnesses or unexplained weakness.

Neuro Hx: Chronic lower back pain for which she is currently undergoing physical therapy. She was evaluated by her primary care physician who did not think any other work-up was necessary at that time (Fig. 41-1).

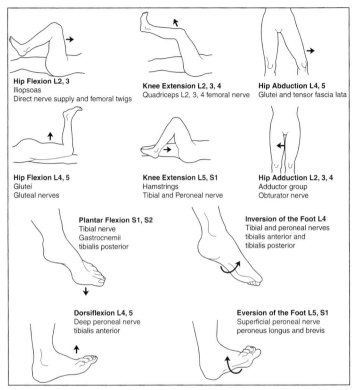

FIGURE **41-1** Leg and foot movements. (*Illustration by Electronic Illustrators Group.*)

THOUGHT QUESTIONS

- Describe the nerves and nerve roots that innervate the major functional muscle groups of the leg.
- Describe the differential diagnosis for a foot drop.
- What are the most common signs and causes of a lumbosacral plexopathy?

A unilateral or asymmetric foot drop (weakness of foot dorsiflexion with or without weakness of other ankle movements) is commonly caused by an L5 radiculopathy, common peroneal nerve palsy, sciatic nerve injury or pyramidal tract lesion (such as multiple sclerosis or following a stroke). Less common causes are motor neuron disease (in adults ALS is the most common) or injury to the lumbosacral plexus involving the L4, L5, and S1 roots, as these are the roots that supply the ankle invertors, evertors, dorsiflexors, and plantar flexors. Symmetrical, bilateral foot drop is usually because of a peripheral polyneuropathy. The temporal course of the onset of her symptoms is of major diagnostic significance. Acute, isolated foot drops are almost always because of an L5 radiculopathy or common peroneal nerve palsy whereas subacute/chronic progressive foot drops are usually because of ALS or a pyramidal lesion.

The characteristic findings in a lumbar plexopathy (formed by the anterior primary rami of spinal nerves L1, L2, L3, and L4) are the combination of weakness in the hip flexors and adductors as well as the knee extensors (muscle groups supplied by the femoral and obturator nerves). Sensory loss over the anteromedial aspect of the thigh and absent or diminished knee jerk are also usually present. The characteristic findings in a sacral plexopathy (formed by the anterior primary rami of spinal nerves L4, L5, S1, S2, and S3) are extensive weakness of the leg and sensory loss in the territories of the peroneal, tibial, and gluteal nerves. The weakness affects the hip extensors and abductors, knee flexors, and ankle dorsi- and plantar flexors. A diminished or absent ankle jerk and numbness over the posterior thigh and calf, anterolateral calf, lateral aspect of the foot and sole are also usually present. Causes of lumbosacral plexopathies include psoas muscle or other intrapelvic hematoma because of bleeding disorders such as hemophilia or anticoagulation, pelvic trauma, abdominal aneurysms, pressure from the head of the infant during prolonged second stage of labor, pelvic neoplasms, postradiation to the pelvis, and vasculitis. In the case of abdominal aneurysms and vasculitis, pain is a common feature.

 CASE CONTINUED

VS:　　Temp 98.6°F BP 110/70 HR 76 RR 16

PE:　　Gen: Unremarkable. No carotid bruits. No lymphadenopathy.

Lungs:　CTA

COR:　　RRR no murmurs. Abdomen: soft, nontender, nondistended, no organomegaly, no bruits. Extremities: no erythema, edema, or tenderness.

Neuro:　CN II–XII: Intact. No dysphagia or dysarthria.

Motor: Normal bulk and tone, no fasciculations. Upper extremities and left leg strength fully intact. Right leg as follows (out of 5): hip flexion, extension, abduction, and adduction, 5; knee flexion and extension, 5; ankle plantar flexion and inversion, 5; ankle dorsiflexion, 2; ankle eversion, 3; and toe extension, 3.

Reflexes: 2+ throughout, no asymmetry noted. Babinski signs absent bilaterally.

Sensory: Slight decrease to light touch and pinprick over the dorsum of the right foot between the big and second toes. Remainder of examination is intact to light touch, pinprick, and vibration.

Coordination: No tremor, dysmetria, or nystagmus

Gait: High steppage gait on right, unable to walk on heels, toe walking intact

 QUESTIONS

41-1. Which nerve root/nerve is affected?
 A. Right common peroneal nerve
 B. Right L5 root lesion
 C. Right L4, L5, S1 plexopathy
 D. Right posterior tibial nerve

41-2. What is the most likely cause of her symptoms?
 A. Pelvic hematoma
 B. Direct pressure to the fibular head
 C. Anterior tibial compartment syndrome
 D. Herniated lumbosacral disc

41-3. What is the most common cause of peripheral neuropathy in the world?
 A. Diabetes
 B. Syphilis
 C. Leprosy
 D. Alcoholism

41-4. Which of the following entrapment neuropathies is seen with equal frequency in nonpregnant versus pregnant patients?
 A. Common peroneal neuropathy
 B. Meralgia paresthetica (lateral femoral cutaneous nerve)
 C. Obturator neuropathy
 D. Femoral neuropathy
 E. Sciatic neuropathy

ANSWERS

41-1. A. The combination of ankle dorsiflexion and eversion weakness with relative sparing of inversion and plantar flexion and minimal sensory loss over the dorsum of the foot is a classic presentation for a common peroneal nerve entrapment. This is the most common entrapment mononeuropathy affecting the lower extremities (the most common in the upper extremities is carpal tunnel syndrome). Although the common peroneal nerve also supplies innervation for inversion and dorsiflexion of the foot and sensation over the anterolateral portion of the lower leg, complete lesions of this nerve are very uncommon. An L5 radiculopathy spares eversion of the foot (this is supplied by S1) and an L4, L5, and S1 plexopathy should affect foot inversion, eversion, plantar, and dorsiflexion relatively equally and is associated with more extensive sensory loss. Entrapment of the posterior tibial nerve (tarsal tunnel syndrome) produces a burning pain on the soles and over the medial aspect of the foot and is associated with intrinsic foot weakness.

41-2. B. The common peroneal nerve is most often damaged as it winds around the neck of the fibula where it is covered only by skin, fat, and fascia. This is most often because of direct pressure from habitual leg crossing, recent weight loss resulting in loss of protective padding, below-the-knee casts, and stretch injuries. The common peroneal nerve can also be compressed by muscle swelling because of excessive exercise, trauma, or ischemia within the anterior tibial compartment. The anterior tibial compartment syndrome is, however, quite painful and associated with lower leg edema. This anatomic distinction is important because recovery from fibular head compression is usually complete using only an ankle-foot orthosis to prevent falls and ankle injuries within three months, and an anterior tibial compartment syndrome usually requires surgical decompression to prevent permanent loss of peroneal nerve function. Given her risk factors of leg crossing and recent weight loss, electrodiagnostic studies to confirm the site of the lesion are usually the only work-up that is needed to make the diagnosis. Further laboratory testing is only indicated if the EMG/NCV studies show more widespread nerve damage or entrapment at a site other than the fibular head. The sciatic nerve splits proximal to the popliteal fossa into the tibial and common peroneal nerves. Even at sites proximal to the splitting of the sciatic nerve (pelvis) the peroneal component is six times as likely to be damaged as the tibial component, often presenting a problem when attempting to localize the lesion. EMG/NCV studies often are necessary to help precisely localize the lesion.

41-3. C. Leprosy is the most common cause of peripheral neuropathies in the world. It predisposes individuals to entrapment neuropathies and often multiple nerves are involved (multiple mononeuropathies). Diabetes and alcoholism cause predominantly axonal peripheral polyneuropathies but also increase vulnerability to entrapment neuropathies.

41-4. A. Pregnancy is a risk factor for several entrapment nerve injuries but not for injury to the common peroneal nerve. Meralgia paresthetica (lateral femoral cutaneous nerve entrapment) produces numbness over the anterior thigh, and is usually entrapped at the level of the inguinal ligament during late pregnancy. Unilateral or bilateral obturator and femoral nerve compression often occur during late pregnancy and delivery because of pressure from the fetal head, forceps, and improperly positioned leg holders. Obturator neuropathies are particularly common during pregnancy, causing severe, intermittent pain in the groin and inner thigh. Femoral neuropathies produce weakened knee extension, a diminished knee jerk reflex, and are usually injured at the time of delivery. Sciatic nerve pain during late pregnancy is also usually because of compression by the fetal head. The most common obstetric palsy is unilateral compression of the lumbosacral trunk (particularly L4 and L5) during a prolonged second stage of labor. Carpal tunnel syndrome is also associated with pregnancy.

 ADDITIONAL SUGGESTED READING

Kim DH, Kline DG. Management and results of peroneal nerve lesions. Neurosurgery 1996;39:312.

Delayed Walking

ID/CC: 28-month-old boy with delayed walking.

HPI: A 28-month-old boy is evaluated for delayed walking. He began taking his first steps with support at 17 months of age, and walking independently after 24 months. His gait is noted to be stiff and awkward by his parents. On review of other development, he achieved "excellent head control" at 8 weeks of age. By 3 months of age, when placed prone, he could hold his head off the bed and extend his neck and look up, which was better than "what his cousins could do at the same age." Since then he has been late in achieving other milestones. His mother also commented that diaper changes are difficult, as he does not like to have his legs splayed and usually cries when she does so. He has a 50-word vocabulary, and attempts to put two words together. He is unable to use a spoon to eat, and still has a rather crude grasp, using all fingers to hold small objects.

PMHx: No other medical problems

Meds: None

All: None

FHx: Noncontributory

SHx: Noncontributory

PE: Weight 12 kg (25th percentile), length: 89 cm (25th percentile). Head circumference 47 cm (<5th percentile). Gen: unremarkable.

Neuro: Mental status: Alert and appropriately interactive

Cranial nerves: Pupils equally reactive. Able to fix and follow objects with eyes.

Face: Symmetric

Motor: Increased muscle tone in all limbs, particularly legs and trunk. Legs would "scissor" when held in axillary suspension. Moved all limbs.

Reflexes: Brisk bilaterally, particularly patellar, with 4 to 5 beats of clonus at ankles.

Plantars: Extensor bilaterally

THOUGHT QUESTIONS

- Where is the lesion (UMN or LMN)?
- What other information will be useful in the differential diagnosis?

The history suggests delay in predominantly motor (gross motor and fine motor) milestones. The infant's examination is notable for increased muscle tone (spasticity) and hyperreflexia. There are numerous signs indicative of spasticity. Passive movement of his limbs demonstrates the hypertonia. When held vertically, suspended from his axillae, his legs "scissor," i.e., adduct at the hips and cross over. This is because of increased muscle tone in the hip adductors commonly seen in children with marked lower extremity spasticity. Similarly, the head control apparently achieved at 8 weeks is not precocious development of head control but rather a sign of hypertonia in neck extensors. The findings on examination indicate a UMN lesion. The presence of microcephaly indicates that the localization is the cerebral cortex. Also, the child's history is one of lack of achieving developmental milestones, as against one of neurologic deterioration, which also factors in to determining the etiology.

Further information that will be useful in the differential diagnosis and in determining the etiology of the child's microcephaly and spastic diapiresis is that pertaining to risk factors for this child for developmental delay. Commonly assessed information includes: details regarding maternal health during pregnancy, gestation at which delivery occurred, complications in the neonatal period, and FHx of neurologic disease.

CASE CONTINUED

Further history was obtained. The child was born at 32 weeks gestation. Preterm labor was because of maternal HTN. He spent 2 weeks in the intensive care nursery, for "routine" issues, including a brief period of mechanical ventilation. A head ultrasound was done in the nursery, which showed a grade 2 intraventricular hemorrhage, which resolved on follow-up scans.

Work-up: An MRI scan of the brain was obtained (Fig. 42-1).

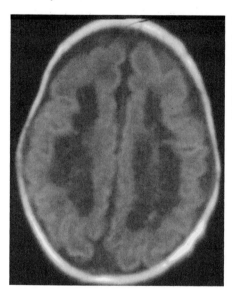

FIGURE 42-1
Axial image of MRI scan of the brain showing periventricular leukomalacia.
(*Image courtesy of Dr J.S. Hahn, Stanford University Medical Center, Stanford, California.*)

THOUGHT QUESTION

■ How does the additional history and magnetic resonance imaging (MRI) scan assist in the differential diagnosis?

Prematurity is a risk factor for developmental delay. Allowance is made for the infant's prematurity while assessing development. As this child was 8 weeks premature, a 2-month allowance would be given for his development. Even with it he is delayed, however. His neonatal course was complicated by an intraventricular hemorrhage, with subsequent periventricular white matter abnormality. The location of the abnormality is anatomically appropriate for the child's findings on examination.

There is no history to suggest maternal infection prior to or early in pregnancy, and no FHx of neurologic illnesses to suggest an inherited neurologic disorder.

The preterm delivery, IVH, and white matter findings on MRI together with predominantly motor delay, microcephaly, and spasticity make it most likely that this is cerebral palsy.

QUESTIONS

42-1. The term "cerebral palsy" implies:
A. Static motor delay
B. Progressive motor delay
C. Isolated cognitive delay
D. Combination of motor and cognitive delay

42-2. Which of the following is a sign of hypotonia rather than spasticity?
A. Scissoring of legs
B. Brisk reflexes
C. Opisthotonos
D. Head lag when pulled to sit

42-3. Grade 2 intraventricular hemorrhage in a newborn implies:
A. Germinal matrix hemorrhage
B. Intraventricular extension of the hemorrhage with ventricular dilatation
C. Intraventricular extension of the hemorrhage without ventricular dilatation
D. Intraparenchymal extension of the hemorrhage

42-4. The following may be used either orally or intrathecally in the chronic treatment of spasticity:
A. Botulinum toxin injections
B. Baclofen
C. Phenobarbital
D. Diazepam

ANSWERS

42-1. A. The term "cerebral palsy" is used to describe a static (nonprogressive) delay in motor skills, usually because of some CNS insult in the perinatal period. In its classic, most pure form, the child's cognitive skills and language are normal or near normal. The classic clinical syndrome is of spastic diplegia or diparesis because of periventricular white matter involvement of predominantly motor fibers to the lower extremities, and was called "Little disease." Progressive motor delay suggests a degenerative condition. Isolated cognitive delay without motor delay would not constitute a diagnosis of cerebral palsy. While some degree of accompanying cognitive delay is often encountered in cerebral palsy, the term really implies motor delay.

42-2. D. Scissoring of legs, brisk deep tendon reflexes and opisthotonos are all signs of increased muscle tone. When an infant is pulled to sit, head lag indicates hypotonia.

42-3. C. On CT, IVH is graded as: grade 1: subependymal hemorrhage without extension, grade 2: subependymal hemorrhage with ventricular extension without ventricular dilatation, grade 3: subependymal hemorrhage with ventricular extension and ventricular dilatation, grade 4: intraparenchymal extension.

42-4. B. Baclofen can be given orally or intrathecally using a surgically implanted baclofen pump. Diazepam is administered orally for treatment of spasticity. Botulinum toxin can be injected into individual muscles periodically to relieve spasticity. Phenobarbital is an anticonvulsant and is not used for treatment of spasticity.

 ADDITIONAL SUGGESTED READING

Ashwal S, Russman BS, Blasco PA, et al. Practice parameter: diagnostic assessment of the child with cerebral palsy: report of the Quality Standards Subcommittee of the American Academy of Neurology and the Practice Committee of the Child Neurology Society. Neurology 2004;62:851.

Yin R, Reddihough D, Ditchfield M, Collins K. Magnetic resonance imaging findings in cerebral palsy. J Paediatr Child Health 2000;36:139.

VII

Patients Who Present with Arm/Hand Weakness, Numbness, or Pain

Bilateral Arm Weakness

ID/CC: 55-year-old woman presents with worsening weakness in her arms.

HPI: AW first noticed slight difficulty putting away dishes in a high cabinet about 3 months ago. Since then she thinks her arms have slowly weakened and she now has trouble blow-drying her hair and putting her makeup on. She has not been dropping things, tripping, or falling. She denies any weakness in her legs but does complain of feeling tired and "weak all over." She used to go for 2-mile walks daily and has had to stop because of her overall fatigue. On neurologic review of systems she complains only of a slight aching sensation in her upper arms. She denies any sensory changes. She has not had any muscle spasms or cramps, headaches, or neck pain. No trouble swallowing. On general review of systems she denies any rashes, fever, weight loss, or night sweats.

PMHx: Multiple miscarriages, environmental allergies

PSHx: Hysterectomy

Meds: St. John's Wort for her fatigue

All: NKDA

SHx: Divorced. No children. Drinks one glass of wine a night. Works full time as a receptionist.

FHx: Patient was adopted. Birth parents are unknown.

Neuro Hx: No prior history of weakness or sensory changes. No history of trauma.

THOUGHT QUESTIONS

- How would you summarize the case thus far?
- Where could her lesion(s) localize? Discuss which ones are more or less likely.
- Describe the nerves and nerve roots that innervate the major functional muscle groups of the arm.

A 55-year-old woman with subacute onset of progressive proximal arm weakness bilaterally in the setting of generalized fatigue. She does not complain of any sensory or lower extremity abnormalities.

Her lesion most likely localizes to the PNS, neuromuscular junction, or muscle. Within the PNS, the lesion could localize to a peripheral polyneuropathy with motor symptoms predominating, bilateral brachial plexopathy, or polyradiculopathy. The symmetrical, proximal onset of weakness makes UMN disease unlikely; as this is usually an asymmetrical process involving proximal and distal antigravity muscles in the upper extremity equally. The proximal onset of weakness also goes against a diagnosis of LMN disease (e.g., ALS). The lack of fluctuating symptoms makes a neuromuscular junction disease (myasthenia gravis) less likely, although not all patients complain of this. The lack of sensory symptoms does not exclude a brachial plexopathy or peripheral polyneuropathy, as many patients do not complain of these particularly when motor symptoms predominate, but does decrease the likelihood.

The major functional muscle groups of the upper extremity (shoulder abduction and adduction, shoulder internal and external rotation, elbow flexion, extension, supination and pronation, wrist extension and flexion, and finger flexion and extension) are supplied by the cervicothoracic roots C5, C6, C7, C8, and T1. These nerve roots intermingle to form the brachial plexus, which gives rise to the axillary, musculocutaneous, radial, median, and ulnar nerves. The suprascapular, subscapular nerves, and the nerve to the latissimus dorsi arise from the proximal trunks of the brachial plexus.

CASE CONTINUED

VS: Temp 98.6°F BP 110/70 HR 74 RR 16

PE: Gen: Patient is obese. No carotid bruits. No lymphadenopathy.

Lungs: CTA. COR: RRR no murmurs

Abdomen: soft, non-tender, non-distended, no organomegaly, no bruits.

Extremities: No erythema, edema, or tenderness

Skin: No rashes.

Neuro: MSE: alert and oriented times 4. Memory and concentration are intact. Affect is appropriate.

CN II–XII: Intact. No dysphagia or dysarthria. No ptosis or other facial weakness

Motor: Muscle bulk and tone are normal. Strength is as follows (out of 5): bilateral latissimus dorsi, deltoid, and supraspinatus, 3; infraspinatus, supraspinatus, and biceps, 4; triceps, wrist extensors, and flexors, 5; finger extensors, and flexors, 5; bilateral hip flexors and extensors, 4; hip abductors and adductors, 5; knee extensors and flexors, 5; plantar and dorsiflexion of foot, 5. Abnormal Gower maneuver. No fatiguing weakness is present.

Reflexes: 1+ throughout. Babinski signs absent bilaterally

Sensory: Intact to light touch, pinprick, temperature, and vibration in all four extremities

Coordination: No tremor, nystagmus, or dysmetria is present.

Gait: Normal. No ataxia, intact tandem, toe and heel gait
(Fig. 43-1)

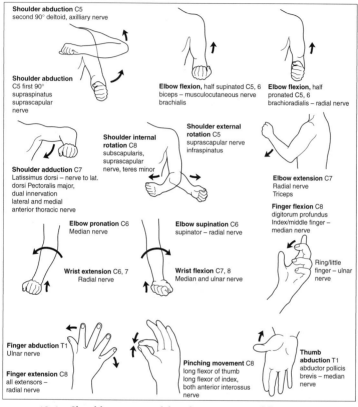

FIGURE 43-1   Shoulder, arm, and hand movements. (*Illustration by Electronic Illustrators Group.*)

Labs: Serum CK: 3,000 mU/mL (upper limit of normal in black women and nonblack men is 345, nonblack women is 145 and black men 520). EMG/NCV show small, polyphasic motor unit action potentials, fibrillations, and increased insertional activity. Nerve conduction amplitudes and velocities are normal. No conduction blocks are present.

Imaging: Chest radiograph, CBC WNL. Stool guaiacs negative.

QUESTIONS

43-1. What is the most likely diagnosis?
- A. Inclusion body myositis (IBM)
- B. Polymyositis
- C. Dermatomyositis
- D. Female carrier of DMD

43-2. What might you expect the muscle biopsy to show?
- A. Rimmed vacuoles and CD8 predominating cellular infiltrate
- B. Variation in fiber size with fibrosis and hyaline fibers
- C. Perifascicular atrophy with CD4 cell predominating infiltrate
- D. Perifascicular atrophy with CD8 cell predominating infiltrate and muscle fiber necrosis

43-3. Which of the following is the standard initial treatment choice?
- A. Prednisone and/or azathioprine
- B. Cyclosporine
- C. Tacrolimus
- D. Riluzole

43-4. Which of the following would suggest an alternate diagnosis?
- A. Collagen vascular diseases
- B. Cardiac conduction defects
- C. Severe muscle pain
- D. Delayed gastric emptying

ANSWERS

43-1. B. With the additional information provided by the PE the lesion most likely localizes to the muscle (myopathy) or less likely to a demyelinating peripheral polyneuropathy. Decreased strength and reflexes out of proportion to the amount of atrophy is consistent with a myopathy or a demyelinating peripheral polyneuropathy. However, the proximal onset of weakness is far more common in myopathic processes than in polyneuropathies and the complete lack of even subtle sensory abnormalities makes a polyneuropathy (or polyradiculoneuropathy) even less likely. The subacute, progressive onset makes an acquired illness rather than a hereditary one more likely.

Polymyositis is an autoimmune disorder in which the muscle fibers are the primary antigenic target. Peak incidence is during childhood or in adults ages 40 to 60 years. It is more common in women than men and usually relapses and remits especially with corticosteroid treatment. It often is accompanied by systemic symptoms such as fever, malaise, and anorexia. The disease begins symmetrically in the proximal musculature and produces marked elevations in CK in the several thousands range.

Dermatomyositis (DM) is also an auto-immune disease with many overlapping clinical features, however a concomitant rash, usually a purple discoloration of the eyelids and cheeks, occurring with the muscular weakness helps distinguish the two. DM occurs more commonly in children than adults.

Ten percent to 20% of patients with adult-onset DM and to a lesser extent, polymyositis, have an underlying malignancy; most commonly stomach, lung, breast, or ovarian carcinoma. Therefore, it is prudent to carry out a chest radiograph, CBC, vaginal examination, and stool guaiacs as screening labs in such patients.

IBM is one of the most common causes of weakness in the elderly but the pattern of weakness often involves finger flexors early in the disease course and although the CK can be somewhat elevated it is usually normal. While some women who carry the mutation in the dystrophin gene on the X chromosome may develop proximal muscle weakness and cardiomyopathy during adulthood, these manifest carriers are very rare, and the symptoms are usually much more slowly progressive.

43-2. D. The pathologic hallmark of polymyositis and dermatomyositis is perifascicular atrophy. In polymyositis, where the primary antigenic target is the muscle, muscle fiber necrosis is also present, whereas in dermatomyositis the primary antigenic target is the vasculature and muscle fiber necrosis is rarely seen. For reasons that are unclear CD8 cellular infiltrates predominate in polymyositis whereas CD4 inflammatory cells predominate in dermatomyositis. Rimmed vacuoles are the characteristic feature on light microscopy for IBM and variation in fiber size and decreased dystrophin staining is what one might expect in a manifest carrier of DMD.

43-3. A. Although well-done blinded, placebo-control trials have not been done, it is the standard of care to treat polymyositis patients with immunosuppressive agents such as prednisone, azathioprine (either alone or in combination) or more recently, IV immunoglobulin (IVIG). Cyclosporine and tacrolimus have shown some efficacy in studies, but are not the standard first-line treatment. Riluzole is an inhibitory of glutamate release used in the treatment of amyotrophic lateral sclerosis.

43-4. C. Polymyositis and dermatomyositis often occur in association with other collagen vascular diseases (the so-called overlap syndromes) and laboratory screening for these should be carried out once the diagnosis has been established. Less commonly poly- and especially dermatomyositis can be associated with carcinomas of the breast, lung, stomach, or ovary. Other tissues involved in poly- and dermatomyositis are cardiac (conduction defects, cardiomyopathy), peripheral vasculature (Raynaud phenomenon), pulmonary (interstitial fibrosis and pneumonitis) and the smooth muscle of the upper gastrointestinal tract (delayed esophageal and gastric emptying). Muscle pain is surprisingly not a symptom of inflammatory myopathies. Some patients complain of annoying, deep muscle aches as this patient does but severe pain strongly points to another diagnosis.

 ADDITIONAL SUGGESTED READING

Lundberg IE. Idiopathic inflammatory myopathies: why do the muscles become weak? Curr Opin Rheumatol 2001;13:457.
Sieb JP, Gillessen T. Iatrogenic and toxic myopathies. Muscle Nerve 2003;7:142.

Neck and Arm Pain

ID/CC: 62-year-old woman with complaint of a sharp stabbing pain in her shoulder radiating down her right arm and into the forearm for 10 weeks

HPI: While cleaning her cupboards, HD developed a sharp stabbing pain in her neck, that she grades as 7 out of 10. The next day the symptoms progressed to include her right shoulder, arm, and forearm. She describes a constant ache in these areas (4 out of 10) with periods of superimposed sharp stabbing pain (7 out of 10). The symptoms are exacerbated by coughing, sneezing, or flexion of the neck. The symptoms have been unrelieved by NSAIDs and 6 weeks of physical therapy.

PMHx: Diabetes mellitus

PSHx: Appendectomy

Meds: Glucophage

All: NKDA

SHx: The patient lives at home with her husband of 40 years.

Habits: No tobacco, history of alcohol abuse—quit 4 years ago, no IVDA or recreational drugs

VS: Temp 99.1°F BP 124/72 HR 80 RR 12

PE/Neuro: The patient has weakness of right elbow flexion (half supinated)—biceps, 4/5. The remainder of the motor examination, including deltoids, triceps, wrist extensors, and hand intrinsics, is intact. There is sensory loss over the thumb and radial border of the hand. There is mild reflex asymmetry, right biceps 1, left biceps 2. Positive Lhermitte sign.

THOUGHT QUESTIONS

- What is the patient's differential diagnosis?
- How would you differentiate between the presence of a peripheral nerve lesion, a root lesion, and a cord lesion?

The patient's symptoms of motor abnormality (weakness of elbow flexion), reflex asymmetry, and sensory loss are consistent with cervical spinal stenosis. The causes include any entity that results in decreased diameter of the cervical spinal canal and includes disc herniation, intraspinal tumor, arachnoiditis, hypertrophy of the lamina or dura, and ossification of the ligaments such as the posterior longitudinal ligament (PLL).

A peripheral nerve lesion may result in either a mononeuropathy or polyneuropathy. A mononeuropathy involves only one peripheral nerve, with minimal sensory loss. In contrast, a polyneuropathy is characterized by a greater degree of sensory loss that is greater distally and may be accompanied by either motor changes and/or reflex abnormalities. A root lesion is distinguished from the above in that the area of involvement is segmental and that pain is the most significant complaint. Weakness, reflex abnormality, and/or atrophy may also be present. The patient's symptoms are consistent with root involvement. A cord lesion involves transverse sensory loss, the level of which depends on the affected level and the specific location on the cord (e.g., anterior cord versus posterior).

CASE CONTINUED

Cervical spine radiographs demonstrate a loss of cervical lordosis. The oblique views demonstrate foraminal encroachment at C5–C6.

While awaiting the MRI, the patient noted weakness in her right arm and increasing difficulty lifting grocery bags. The pain also increased significantly to 9 out of 10 in intensity and began to interfere with her activities of daily living.

The MRI demonstrates a herniation of the intervertebral disc at C5/6. The disc material is eccentric to the right and impinges the C6 nerve root.

THOUGHT QUESTIONS

- What are key components of radiculopathy?
- Differentiate between the terms spondylosis, spondylolisthesis, and spondylolysis.

The term radiculopathy refers to symptoms resulting from compression of adjacent nerve root by any of a variety of causes including disc protrusion and osteophytes. The resulting clinical features include pain and paresthesias, sensory loss, muscle weakness, and reflex impairment.

Spondylosis refers to a nonspecific degenerative process of the spine. In the case of the cervical spine, the term cervical stenosis is used synonymously with cervical spondylosis. Spondylolisthesis describes anterior subluxation of one vertebral body on another. The term spondylolysis is used as an alternative term for isthmic spondylolisthesis, a defect in the pars interarticularis.

CASE CONTINUED

The patient is scheduled for anterior cervical discectomy with fusion (ACDF).

QUESTIONS

44-1. Which of the following muscles is involved with a nerve root lesion at C6?
- A. Deltoid
- B. Biceps
- C. Triceps
- D. Wrist extensors

44-2. What reflex is associated with C5–C6?
- A. Cremasteric reflex
- B. Quadriceps
- C. Triceps
- D. Biceps

44-3. Which of the following describes Lhermitte's sign?
   A. Weakness and atrophy of the hands
   B. Electric shock-like sensations radiating down the back with neck flexion
   C. Diminished lower extremity reflexes
   D. Motor weakness in bilateral upper extremities

44-4. Which of the following MRI findings would be an indication for surgical intervention?
   A. Disc herniation at C4/5
   B. Disc herniation at C5/6
   C. Disc herniation at C6/7
   D. None of the above

ANSWERS

44-1. B. A motor deficit of the deltoid muscle results from a C5 root lesion. Weakness of the triceps muscle and wrist extensors result from a root lesion of C7. Biceps weakness results from a root lesion of C6.

44-2. D. The biceps reflex is most closely associated with C5/6. The cremasteric reflex is associated with L2/3, the quadriceps reflex is associated with L3/4, and the triceps reflex is associated with C6/7.

44-3. B. Lhermitte's sign describes the symptom of electric shock-like sensation radiating down the back of the patient, produced by neck flexion. It is useful as a clinical symptom in the evaluation of cervical radiculopathy. It is however nonspecific, and may be found in a variety of clinical conditions including cervical disc herniation, multiple sclerosis, and Chiari I malformation.

44-4. D. The radiographic finding of intervertebral disc herniation in and of itself is not an indication for surgical intervention. The clinical findings of acute cervical radiculopathy resulting from a disc herniation will recover without surgical intervention in the majority of patients. Greater than 90% will recover with conservative management alone. Surgery is indicated when these measures fail to improve the patient's symptoms or if there is progressive neurologic deficit while being managed conservatively.

ADDITIONAL SUGGESTED READING

Kasch H, Bach FW, Stengaard-Pedersen K, Jensen TS. Development in pain and neurologic complaints after whiplash: A 1-year prospective study. Neurology 2003;60:743.

Stiell IG, Clement CM, McKnight RD, et al. The Canadian C-spine rule versus the NEXUS low-risk criteria in patients with trauma. N Engl J Med 2003;349:2510.

Infant not Moving Right Arm

CC/ID: Newborn female with no movement of her right arm

HPI: Baby NP was a few hours old when the nurses caring for her noticed that she wasn't moving her right arm. She was born at term to a G3P2 woman, with good prenatal care and no pregnancy complications. Labor was prolonged, and was complicated by shoulder dystocia. The baby was born vaginally, and weighed 4 kg. She was admitted for observation to the neonatal intensive care unit (NICU) for tachypnea. At 4 hours of life, the nurse checking her noticed that her right arm was not moving and was flaccid. She brings this to the attention of NICU resident.

PMHx:	As above
Meds:	Ampicillin, gentamicin, IV fluids
All:	None
FHx:	Unremarkable
SHx:	Two older siblings, both healthy
PE:	Gen: Caput succedaneum, some facial bruising
CV:	No murmur
Lungs:	Clear
Abdomen:	No organomegaly
Skin:	1 café-au-lait spot on buttock
Spine:	Normal
Neuro:	Alert, cries during examination
Cranial nerves:	Intact

Motor: Normal tone, reflexes, and movements in lower extremities and left upper extremity

Right upper
extremity: Flaccid, with arm held internally rotated at the shoulder and pronated at the elbow. No spontaneous movement at the shoulder. No elbow flexion, a flicker of elbow extension seen. Able to grasp finger. Biceps reflex absent, triceps present. Winces in response to tactile stimulation of arm.

VS: WNL

THOUGHT QUESTIONS

- Where does this lesion most likely localize?
- What additional tests will help in the differential diagnosis?

The key finding on examination of baby NP is a flaccid paresis of the right upper extremity. Although detailed muscle strength testing is difficult in a newborn, the baby's examination suggests a predominantly proximal weakness, with shoulder and biceps affected to the greatest extent. Findings are suggestive of a LMN lesion.

Possibilities to be considered in localizing the lesion are a lesion involving the left cerebral hemisphere. Upper-extremity weakness would be possible with a left middle cerebral artery distribution lesion, but isolated arm weakness without facial involvement would be unusual. Similarly, lesions in the internal capsule or lower down in the brainstem are capable of causing arm weakness, but produce a wider range of deficits.

Further down the neuraxis, a spinal cord lesion could produce a flaccid monoparesis, but the weakness is likely to be uniform throughout the limb. Even more distally a lesion involving the spinal nerve roots should be considered, in which case sensory findings should be expected (not easy to test in a newborn!). Brachial plexus lesions can produce weakness as described here. The pattern of weakness involves muscles innervated by roots C5 and C6, which form the upper portion of the brachial plexus. This would also explain the absent biceps reflex, which has a spinal root level of C5–C6.

Thinking and working one's way through the possibilities and correlating them with the infant's examination localizes the lesion to the brachial plexus. The infant's birth history is notable for shoulder dystocia, which is a recognized risk factor for traction on the brachial plexus during a difficult delivery.

When the history is obvious, and the infant's examination correlates with a brachial plexus injury, further diagnostic work-up may not be necessary. A nerve conduction study may aid in confirming the diagnosis, but these tests are very difficult to perform and interpret in a newborn and add little to the picture.

 ## CASE CONTINUED

NP was observed for the next few days. By day three of life, there was a little spontaneous movement in her arm, a flicker of flexion at the elbow and at the shoulder. Her arm was still flaccid and the biceps reflex absent. She remained alert, made good eye contact, fed well, and was discharged to home. Physical therapy was advised as an outpatient.

At follow-up 3 months later, her exam showed improved right upper extremity function. She was able to lift her arm against gravity, and had started reaching out for her mobile. Elbow flexion was nearly normal, and the biceps reflex, although still hypoactive, was now elicitable.

 ## THOUGHT QUESTION

■ How does this course influence the previously made diagnosis?

This course is typical for a brachial plexus injury at birth. The usual pathophysiology is traction on the nerve resulting in a neurapraxia, which gradually gets better over time. Physical therapy helps in maintaining range of motion of the shoulder and elbow, and prevents contractures or joint stiffness.

In severe cases, where there may have been actual avulsion of nerve roots, recovery does not follow this course, and surgical treatment may be necessary.

QUESTIONS

45-1. This baby has:
   A. Erb palsy
   B. Klumpke palsy
   C. Neither
   D. Both

45-2. The spinal cord root level of the triceps reflex is:
   A. C8–T1
   B. C7–C8
   C. C6,7,8
   D. C5,6

45-3. The posterior cord of the brachial plexus forms which of the following nerves:
   A. Ulnar nerve
   B. Median nerve
   C. Radial nerve
   D. Musculocutaneous nerve

45-4. The characteristic position of the upper extremity in Erb palsy is called:
   A. Nursemaid elbow
   B. Waiter's tip hand
   C. Claw hand
   D. None of the above

ANSWERS

45-1. A. The clinical picture produced by lesions involving the upper trunk of the brachial plexus (spinal roots C5,6, sometimes 7) is called Erb palsy. Klumpke palsy is also caused by lesions in the brachial plexus, involving the lower trunk of the brachial plexus (spinal roots C8–T1).

45-2. C. The spinal cord root level of the commonly elicited muscle stretch reflexes are: biceps: C5,6; brachioradialis: C5,6; triceps: C6,7,8; patellar: L2,3,4; tendo Achilles: S1,S2.

45-3. C. The median nerve is derived from the lateral and medial cords of the brachial plexus. The ulnar nerve is derived from the medial cord. The musculocutaneous nerve is derived from the lateral cord. The radial nerve is derived from the posterior cord of the brachial plexus.

45-4. B. The characteristic position of the upper extremity in Erb palsy is called "waiter's tip hand." The position comprises adduction and internal rotation at the shoulder, extension and pronation at the elbow, and partial flexion of the wrist. Claw hand is characteristic of lesions involving the lower trunk of the brachial plexus. Nursemaid elbow is subluxation of the radial head because of trauma.

 ADDITIONAL SUGGESTED READING

ACOG practice bulletin clinical management guidelines for obstetrician-gynecologists. Shoulder dystocia. Obstet Gynecol 2002;100:1045.

Right Hand Weakness

   ID/CC: 53-year-old right-handed man presents with progressive right-hand weakness

HPI: About 8 months ago ML began occasionally dropping things with his right hand. Gradually, he noticed a deterioration in his handwriting and he began to lose grip strength. He also complains of painful cramping in both hands at night, more pronounced on the right. He denies any sensory changes or paresthesias; head, neck, or shoulder pain; or any recent injuries. There is no diurnal variation to his hand weakness.

PMHx: Chronic lower back pain following an injury 20 years ago

PSHx: S/P L4–L5 lumbar laminectomy 10 years prior

Meds: Ibuprofen 600 mg as needed

All: NKDA

SHx: Engineer, married with two children. Does not smoke or drink alcohol.

FHx: Grandmother who died of advanced Parkinson's disease

Neuro Hx: No history of tremor, memory loss, or head injury

THOUGHT QUESTIONS

- Where could his lesion(s) localize? (at least five possibilities)
- What signs will you look for on examination to aid in localization?
- What is an EMG and how can it be useful in aiding in localization?

Weakness in the right hand can be caused by a lesion affecting: (1) UMNs and their pathways (left motor cortex, left internal capsule, left pyramidal tract decussation in the medulla to the right lateral corticospinal tract in the spinal cord above the level of C7/C8); (2) LMNs at C7/C8 either from intrinsic cord lesions or diseases affecting alpha motor neurons of the spinal cord; (3) nerve roots as they exit the spinal cord or the proximal brachial plexus; (4) peripheral nerves; (5) neuromuscular junction (NMJ); and (6) muscles. The chronic progression of his symptoms suggests a degenerative process or slow-growing mass. The lack of sensory symptoms makes a peripheral nerve process less likely; however, there are a variety of rare, pure motor neuropathies that could present in such a manner.

The most important signs to look for on PE are UMN signs, LMN signs, and sensory involvement. UMN signs include paresis or paralysis, limb spasticity, hyperreflexia, extensor plantar responses (Babinski sign), brisk jaw jerk, clonus, and decreased superficial cutaneous reflexes (abdominal, corneal, and cremesteric). LMN signs include focal or multifocal weakness or paralysis, hypotonia, hyporeflexia, atrophy, muscle fasciculation (detectable by the naked eye), and fibrillations (detectable by EMG). Stiffness, which can be painful, is a common symptom of UMN disease, while cramping is a common complaint in LMN disease.

An EMG measures the electrical characteristics of muscle groups at the site of insertion of the needle at rest and following electrical stimulation. An EMG is able to detect abnormalities in the amplitude, frequency, and phasic response of compound muscle action potentials (CMAPs) and abnormalities of resting muscle such as increased insertional activity, fibrillations, and positive sharp waves. An EMG can usually distinguish between: (1) myopathies (primary muscle disorders), (2) myotonic disorders, (3) NMJ disorders, and (4) disorders that lead to denervation of muscle (nerve, root, or α-motor neuron diseases). Myopathies show reduced amplitude CMAPs and a variable amount of increased insertional activity and complex polyphasic motor unit potentials. An EMG is not useful in distinguishing between the different types of myopathies except for those associated with myotonia. Denervation produces polyphasic action potentials, positive sharp waves, bizarre high frequency discharges, fibrillations, and fasciculations. NMJ disorders (myasthenia gravis, Lambert-Eaton myasthenic syndrome, and botulism) usually show normal resting and brief stimulation responses but demonstrate characteristic abnormalities following repetitive stimulation of the same muscle group.

CASE CONTINUED

VS: Temp 98.6°F BP 110/70 HR 76

PE: Gen: Unremarkable. No carotid bruits. No lymphadenopathy. Lungs: CTA. COR: RRR no murmurs. Abdomen: Soft, nontender, nondistended, no organomegaly.

Neuro: MSE: 30/30 MMSE. CN II–XII: intact. No dysphagia, dysarthria, or tongue weakness or fasciculations.

Motor: Right hand strength 3/5, left hand 4/5. Right biceps and triceps 4/5. Remainder of individual muscle group testing 5/5 strength. Atrophy of intrinsic right hand muscles with fasciculations. Fasciculations in left hand and right quadriceps as well.

Reflexes: 3+ bilateral upper extremities. 2+ bilateral lower extremities. Extensor plantar response on right.

Sensory: Intact to light touch, pinprick, vibration, and temperature in all four extremities

Coordination: No dysmetria, tremor, or nystagmus

Gait: Normal, no ataxia, and intact tandem gait

QUESTIONS

46-1. What is the most likely diagnosis?
  A. CIDP
  B. ALS
  C. Cervical cord lesion
  D. Muscular dystrophy
  E. None of the above

46-2. What work-up should be ordered?
  A. Muscle and nerve biopsy
  B. Brain and cervical spine MRI
  C. CK
  D. All of the above

46-3. What will the EMG and NCV most likely show?
   A. Widespread denervation with fibrillation and fasciculation potentials, and positive waves. Normal or near normal NCV.
   B. CMAP with a 15% decremental response to repetitive nerve stimulation. Normal or near normal NCV.
   C. Widespread denervation with fibrillation and fasciculation potentials and positive waves. Low CMAP with abnormal temporal dispersion. NCV with multiple sites of conduction block at nonentrapment sites.
   D. Multifocal denervation with fibrillation and fasciculation potentials. NCV show reduction of motor nerve conduction velocities below 70% of normal, conduction block in several motor nerves, and absent F-waves.

46-4. What is his prognosis?
   A. Excellent given appropriate therapy is initiated promptly
   B. 5-year survival 5%
   C. 5-year survival 40%
   D. 5-year survival 25%

ANSWERS

46-1. B. ALS is the most likely diagnosis given the patient's history and examination findings. The peak age of onset of ALS is in the sixth decade and it is slightly more common in men than women. In most cases it is sporadic, although 5% to 10% of cases are familial. ALS is subdivided clinically into two categories based on the site of onset of the disease, either in the limbs or in the bulbar muscles. Onset in the bulbar muscles (dysphagia, dysarthria, and difficulty in mastication) has a more rapidly progressive course, although almost all patients with the limb onset form will eventually develop bulbar dysfunction. Respiratory failure and related complications is usually the final cause of death. The disease is characterized by the presence of both UMN and LMN signs and should be suspected in anyone with weakness and atrophy with preserved or increased reflexes. ALS is caused by the progressive loss of α motor neurons in the brainstem and spinal cord and atrophy of the frontal precentral gyrus (motor cortex).

46-2. C. The diagnosis of ALS is confirmed simply by an EMG, NCV, and CK. CK is elevated in 35% to 70% of patients with ALS and, while not specific, helps exclude other diseases on the differential diagnosis such as pure UMN lesions. Rarely, an ALS-like syndrome can occur in the setting of thyroid disease, B12 deficiency, hexosaminidase A deficiency (in young people), postpolio syndrome, dysproteinemia, and lead toxicity and therefore, these illnesses should be screened for in the initial work-up, particularly in unusual cases.

46-3. A. Although decremental responses with repetitive stimulation can be seen in ALS and are associated with a poorer prognosis, it rarely reaches 15%, which is diagnostic for myasthenia gravis. Widespread denervation (at least three limbs) with a low CMAP and occasional giant action potentials are the characteristic findings in ALS. The NCVs are usually normal although occasionally a slight prolongation of F-wave latency and abnormal sural nerve conduction can be seen. A rare but important treatable neuropathy that can mimic ALS is multifocal motor neuropathy (MMN) with conduction block. In this disease, the EMG is very similar to ALS but the NCVs show multiple sites of conduction block along motor nerves at nonentrapment sites. The pattern of EMG evidence of denervation and reinnervation accompanied by absent F waves and multiple conduction blocks and markedly diminished conduction velocities in motor nerves are the typical findings in CIDP.

46-4. D. The 5-year survival rate for patients with sporadic, limb-onset ALS is 25%.

 ADDITIONAL SUGGESTED READING

Kaufmann P, Pullman SL, Shungu DC, et al. Objective tests for upper motor neuron involvement in amyotrophic lateral sclerosis (ALS). Neurology 2004;62:1753.

Rowland, LP, Shneider, NA. Amyotrophic lateral sclerosis. N Engl J Med 2001;344:1688.

Acute Right Arm Weakness and Neck Pain

ID/CC: 47-year-old woman with acute right arm weakness and neck pain

HPI: One day prior, KS developed a pain in the left side of her neck and noticed that her left eyelid was droopy. She then developed a left temporal headache, and decided to go to bed to sleep it off. She awoke this morning and noted that her right arm was weak. Her husband noticed that her right face was drooping. When he asked her what was wrong, he noted that she had some difficulty explaining to him but he was able to understand what she meant. He called 911, and she was brought to the emergency room 1 hour later. At the time of your evaluation, KS thinks her arm is getting better, and her husband reports that her speech sounds more normal. She still has left-sided neck pain and headache.

PMHx: HTN, depression

PSHx: C-section 15 years prior

Meds: Hydrochlorothiazide (HCTZ), sertraline

All: NKDA

FHx: No history of strokes, aneurysms, or clotting disorder

SHx: Married mother of one child. Works as a computer analyst.

Habits: Smokes one half PPD, occasional alcohol, no IVDA or recreational drugs

THOUGHT QUESTIONS

- What is the differential diagnosis?
- Is this patient a candidate for acute intervention, i.e., thrombolysis?

The most obvious and most urgent possible cause of the patient's symptoms is a stroke. The pattern of deficits is most consistent with an acute ischemic infarct. Intracerebral hemorrhages tend to have less respect for vascular territories, but this possibility should be ruled out with a noncontrast head CT nonetheless. Causes of ischemic stroke include cardioembolic, small-vessel in situ thrombosis, artery-artery embolus, and large vessel in situ thrombosis.

In the evaluation of an acute ischemic stroke, it is important to establish quickly whether the patient is a candidate for thrombolysis with IV tissue plasminogen activator (t-PA). One requirement is a maximum time period of 3 hours between onset of symptoms and administration of t-PA. While this patient presents to the emergency room within 1 hour of noticing her symptoms, she could have developed them in her sleep. In cases where the patient awakes with symptoms or is found with symptoms and unable to tell what time they started, the time of onset is by default the time the patient was last seen normal. Another important criterion for thrombolysis is whether the symptoms are improving. Given the risks of bleeding complications, t-PA guidelines dictate that, in patients who are improving, the potential benefits of IV t-PA are outweighed by the risks of bleeding. In this case, KS is not a candidate for thrombolysis given her unclear time of onset and her improving symptoms. While acute stroke is always an urgent matter, the expediency of work-up becomes more imperative when the patient is being considered for thrombolysis.

CASE CONTINUED

VS: Temp 98.1°F BP 155/80 HR 78 RR 16

PE: No carotid bruits, regular cardiac rhythm, no rashes or petechiae

Neuro: Mental status reveals some slight hesitancy of speech with short phrases, but intact comprehension, naming, and repetition.

Cranial nerve exam is notable for anisocoria, with right pupil 1 mm larger than left, although both pupils react to light. The anisocoria is increased in dark light. She also has a ptosis of the left upper eyelid, and a mild UMN pattern right facial droop. Motor testing reveals a right pronator drift and 4/5 right upper extremity weakness. Right lower extremity is full strength. Sensory, reflex, coordination, and gait are all WNL.

Labs/drug screen: WNL

THOUGHT QUESTIONS

- What is the most likely cause of the patient's symptoms?
- What neuroimaging would you obtain to confirm your diagnosis?

In addition to a transcortical motor aphasia and right face and arm weakness, the patient has a left Horner's syndrome, with left eyelid ptosis and left pupil miosis. This constellation is worrisome for a left carotid artery dissection. The superior cervical sympathetic fibers course along the internal carotid artery as they pass from the neck into the cranial vault. Any lesion that exerts mass effect in the vicinity of the sympathetic fibers can cause a deficit of sympathetic outflow to the pupillodilator and the levator palpebrae superioris muscles, with resultant unopposed parasympathetic stimulation. In classic Horner's syndrome, there is also anhidrosis of the ipsilateral forehead as sympathetic innervation of the sweat glands is disrupted as it courses along the common carotid and then external carotid artery. Neck pain is sometimes associated with carotid or vertebral artery dissection. The mechanism by which cranial arterial dissections are thought to cause infarction is local thrombogenesis at the site of endothelial damage, leading to pieces of clot that embolize and travel "downstream" to the smaller intracranial arteries. While carotid and vertebral artery dissections are an uncommon cause of stroke overall, they are an important cause of ischemic stroke in young and middle-aged persons.

A CT scan is fast and inexpensive, and can show hemorrhage or large infarctions. While CT scans may reveal a hypodensity at the site of an infarction, these changes are often not apparent early in the course of infarction. MRI with diffusion-weighted imaging is more sensitive for acute infarction and gives better resolution of the precise area affected. While conventional angiography is the gold standard for detecting dissection, CT angiography and MR angiography (MRA) are both useful in detecting sites of intracranial vessel stenosis, including carotid dissection, and are less invasive and more readily available in the acute setting. A classic sign of dissection on angiography is a "flame sign," a bulge in the artery, which then tapers off like a flame. If dissection is suspected, the radiologist should be made aware as there are special techniques employed to maximize resolution of possible arterial lesions.

 CASE CONTINUED

MRI reveals a diffusion abnormality in the left frontal area, in the vicinity of the motor cortex. MRA reveals a focal dilatation with a false lumen in the internal carotid artery and severe stenosis at the site of dissection. The patient is admitted to the hospital for further care.

 QUESTIONS

47-1. What risk factors are associated with carotid or vertebral artery dissection?
   A. Genetic connective tissue disorders
   B. Recent respiratory tract infection
   C. Chiropractic neck manipulation
   D. All of the above

47-2. Which vascular territory is most likely involved in the above case?
   A. Left middle cerebral artery (MCA) inferior branch
   B. Left MCA superior branch
   C. Left anterior cerebral artery (ACA), or
   D. Left posterior cerebral artery (PCA)

47-3. What signs would be expected in a left vertebral artery dissection?
   A. Frontal headache
   B. Dysarthria
   C. Ataxia
   D. All of the above

47-4. What is the standard treatment for acute carotid artery dissection?
- A. Carotid endarterectomy
- B. Tight BP control
- C. Anti-coagulation with heparin and then warfarin sodium (Coumadin) for 3 to 6 months
- D. None of the above

ANSWERS

47-1. D. Spontaneous dissections of both carotid and vertebral arteries are thought to be associated with defects in the arterial wall. A small percentage of patients have defined connective tissue disorders such as Ehlers-Danlos's syndrome or Marfan's syndrome, but a much larger percentage are felt to have an unnamed connective tissue disorder. Environmental factors associated with spontaneous dissections of the carotid and vertebral arteries include hyperextension or rotation of the neck (yoga, painting a ceiling, coughing, etc.), chiropractic manipulation of the neck (vertebral > carotid dissection), and recent history of respiratory tract infection.

47-2. B. The left MCA superior branch supplies the Broca area and the motor cortex for the face and arm.

47-3. D. Local signs of vertebral artery dissection include pain in the back of the neck, occipital and sometimes frontal headache. Ischemic symptoms in the posterior circulation include brainstem, cerebellar, and posterior cerebral functions.

47-4. C. The mechanism of infarct in 90% of dissections is embolic, and treatment with anti-coagulation initially with heparin and then warfarin sodium (Coumadin) for a period of 3 to 6 months is the standard treatment. In cases where anti-coagulation is too risky or symptoms are mild, antiplatelet agents such as aspirin or clopidogrel bisulfate (Plavix) are sometimes used. Surgical or endovascular procedures are risky because of the vascular defects, but are sometimes used in cases of recurrent infarcts despite anti-coagulation. Unlike aortic dissections which tend to rupture or extend and require aggressive BP control, carotid dissections never rupture and rarely extend past the small osseous foramen through which the artery enters the cranial vault.

ADDITIONAL SUGGESTED READING

Schievink W. Spontaneous dissection of the carotid and vertebral arteries. N Engl J Med 2001;344:898–906.

Right-Hand Numbness

ID/CC: A 48-year-old right-handed female presents with numb right hand.

HPI: CT is a 48-year-old right-handed female with the chief complaint of numbness and weakness in her right hand. Her symptoms began 2 years ago, with mild numbness intermittently in her right hand. The numbness was most apparent while working at her computer, or upon awakening. Typically, shaking her hand (as if shaking water off her hand) made the numbness go away. Otherwise, the numbness would improve and disappear altogether with rest. Over 2 years the numbness became more apparent to the patient and more frequent; it was noticeable while driving, cutting vegetables, and at other times. At times she would wake up at night with her right hand numb and hand and forearm sore. In the month prior to seeking medical attention, she noticed some clumsiness in her right hand.

PMH: Mitral valve prolapse

PSH: Caesarean section times 2

Meds: None

All: Penicillin

FHx: Diabetes mellitus in the patient's mother

SHx: Nonsmoker, occasionally drinks wine. Works as an administrative assistant.

PE: Gen: normal

VS: Normal

Neuro: Mental status: normal. Cranial nerves: normal.

Motor: UE: 5/5 strength in deltoid, biceps, triceps, wrist extensors and flexors. Weakness in right thumb abduction and opposition. Remainder of strength testing normal. Atrophy of thenar eminence. Sustained flexion of the wrists reproduces the patient's symptoms.

Reflexes: Normal

Sensory examination: Decreased pinprick over palmar aspect of right thumb, index and middle finger

Gait and coordination: Normal

THOUGHT QUESTION

- ■ Where is the lesion?

The key findings in this case are chronic progressive numbness over time, a focal predominantly sensory deficit, and minimal motor weakness.

In the neuraxis, a lesion such as a small stroke in the thalamus can produce contralateral sensory symptoms, but the symptoms are more likely to be persistent rather than intermittent and less likely to affect as restricted an area. Lesions in the sensory cortex could also produce hand paresthesias; again a broader region is more likely to be affected.

Lesions affecting the spinal roots such as C6 or C7 cause sensory symptoms in the hand, but accompanying pain is a common finding. Also usually such radiculopathies produce some weakness in muscles innervated by those roots, and reflexes may be depressed. Symptoms being worse at night is also unusual for a radiculopathy.

Lesion in an individual nerve could cause symptoms as described above. Compressive lesions, or entrapment of the nerve, are likely to produce such symptoms. The median nerve provides sensory innervation to the medial fingers of the hand, and has some motor innervation to intrinsic hand muscles as well, and is a likely location as to where the lesion is.

Often the PE, particularly a careful motor examination (paying attention to intrinsic muscles in the hand) and sensory examination of the hand will show a pattern consistent with a median nerve lesion. Electrodiagnostic studies (nerve conduction studies and electromyography) can also be helpful in the differential diagnosis.

CASE CONTINUED

Labs: CBC: WNL. Chemistries: WNL.

A nerve conduction study is obtained. It shows decreased conduction velocity in the median nerve of the right hand.

THOUGHT QUESTIONS

- What is the diagnosis?
- What is Tinel sign?

The patient's history and examination alert one to the high likelihood of this being a median nerve process. The electrodiagnostic study confirms this. The diagnosis is a chronic entrapment neuropathy of the median nerve at the wrist, called carpal tunnel syndrome.

Tinel sign is a finding on examination. Light percussion over the volar aspect of the wrist, over the flexor retinaculum causes numbness in the hand. Other provocative maneuvers that reproduce median nerve compression symptoms are:

Phalen sign: sustained hyperflexion of the wrists causes hand weakness in a median nerve distribution pattern (demonstrated in this patient).

Tourniquet test: tying a tourniquet proximal to the wrist causes typical hand numbness.

QUESTIONS

48-1. Carpal tunnel syndrome is associated with which of the following conditions?
- A. Hypothyroidism
- B. Pregnancy
- C. Diabetes mellitus
- D. All of the above

48-2. Motor weakness in carpal tunnel syndrome is:
- A. Often the presenting sign
- B. Necessarily present for diagnosis
- C. Seen late in the course of the disease
- D. Seen in isolation

48-3. Treatment of carpal tunnel syndrome includes which of the following?
- A. Splinting the wrist
- B. Local corticosteroid injection
- C. Surgical division of the flexor retinaculum
- D. NSAIDs
- E. All of the above

48-4. Sensory supply to the dorsal aspect of the hand comes from which nerve?
- A. Median nerve
- B. Radial nerve
- C. Ulnar nerve
- D. None of the above
- E. All of the above

 ANSWERS

48-1. D. Hypothyroidism is believed to cause carpal tunnel syndrome because of deposition of myxedematous material in the carpal tunnel. The exact reason for its developing in pregnancy and diabetes is unclear (Table 48-1).

TABLE **48-1** Conditions Associated with Carpal Tunnel Syndrome

Endocrine Disorders
Diabetes mellitus
Hypothyroidism
Acromegaly
Pregnancy
Obesity
Connective Tissue Disorders
Rheumatoid arthritis
Amyloidosis
Granulomatous diseases
Sarcoidosis
Tuberculosis
Tenosynovitis
Trauma (such as fractures)
Space-occupying lesions
Idiopathic

48-2. C. Carpal tunnel syndrome commonly presents with sensory symptoms in the hand. Classic distribution of numbness is in medial nerve distribution, i.e., involving palmar aspect on thumb, index finger, middle finger, and radial half of ring finger. Not all patients can describe numbness with such precision, and will often complain of numbness in the tips of the fingers. Evolution of symptoms as described in this case is quite typical. Weakness and atrophy over the abductor pollicis brevis are findings late in the disease course.

48-3. E. Nonsurgical treatment is recommended in early and mild cases of carpal tunnel syndrome. These conservative measures include: (1) avoidance of activities that exacerbate symptoms, (2) splinting the wrist, (3) NSAIDs, and (4) local injections of steroids. If an underlying cause is identified, treatment of the etiologic factor is also advised. Failure of nonsurgical measures and progressive thenar atrophy are indications to pursue a surgical treatment. Surgical division of the flexor retinaculum is the definitive treatment for the condition, and is performed as an open procedure or endoscopically.

48-4. B. The median and ulnar nerves provide sensory innervation for the palm. Sensory supply to the dorsal aspect of the hand comes from the radial nerve.

 ADDITIONAL SUGGESTED READING

D'Arcy CA, McGee S. The rational clinical examination. Does this patient have carpal tunnel syndrome? JAMA 2000;283:3110.

VIII

Patients Who Present with Sleep and Speech Problems

Excessive Daytime Sleepiness

ID/CC: 36-year-old man presents to your office complaining of worsening fatigue over the last several years.

HPI: Over the last 6 years SD complains that he has become increasingly tired during the day, requiring frequent naps. He wakes up feeling better, but still tired. He originally attributed it to "getting old" and being "out of shape." He has gained 40 pounds over the last 6 years. Over the last year he has fallen asleep at work unexpectedly several times and is in jeopardy of losing his job. He also complains of "memory problems," particularly when starting new projects at work. He says he is unable to learn new things. He has also been having marital trouble because of his increasing irritability. His wife tells him that he is a restless sleeper and wheezes a lot during his sleep, for which he underwent an asthma evaluation several years ago that was negative. They have slept in separate beds for several years now because of this. The patient is not aware of any of his nocturnal sleep disturbances. SD denies insomnia, and says he sleeps on average eight to nine hours a night. On neurologic review of systems he also complains of several episodes of enuresis over the last year.

PMHx: None

PSHx: Appendectomy at age 8

Meds: None

All: NKDA

SHx: Married for 6 years, with two children, works as an engineer for a high-tech company. He does not drink or smoke.

FHx: No history of sleep disorders or neurodegenerative conditions

Neuro Hx: No history of seizures, blackouts, or head injury

THOUGHT QUESTIONS

- How would you summarize the case thus far?
- What is the differential diagnosis?
- What are the clinical characteristics of narcolepsy?

A middle-aged man with chronic excessive daytime sleepiness accompanied more recently by memory problems, irritability, and enuresis. It is important to distinguish excessive daytime sleepiness from insomnia as excessive daytime sleepiness is usually because of an organic cause whereas insomnia is usually secondary to psychologic or psychiatric causes. Poor concentration (often reported as memory problems by patients), irritability, feeling sad, and a general lack of interest are all symptoms commonly reported in patients with chronic sleep deprivation and patients with excessive daytime sleepiness without insomnia.

The differential diagnosis for excessive daytime sleepiness in the absence of insomnia includes (1) drugs and alcohol, particularly sedatives, sympathomimetic drugs, and β-blockers; (2) narcolepsy; (3) sleep apnea: obstructive, central, or mixed; (4) sleep-related motor disorders such as restless legs syndrome, sleep myoclonus, bruxism, hypnic jerks, and frequent sleep arousals; (5) endocrine/metabolic causes such as hypoglycemia, anemia, hepatic encephalopathy, uremia, and left ventricular failure; (6) depression: hypersomnia is a symptom in 20% of depressed patients, particularly those with bipolar illness; (7) neurodegenerative illnesses such as Alzheimer's disease, multiple sclerosis, Parkinson's disease, and multi-infarct dementia.

While enuresis can occur in conjunction with parasomnias (rapid eye movement [REM]-sleep behavior disorder, nightmares, and sleep terrors) and chronic obstructive sleep apnea, it can also be caused by epilepsy.

Narcolepsy is a primary sleep disorder characterized by excessive daytime sleepiness and frequent sleep attacks during the daytime accompanied by cataplexy. Cataplexy is defined as the sudden loss of postural tone while still conscious, usually brought on by intense emotions such as laughter or fear. Other features of narcolepsy include sleep paralysis (total paralysis usually lasting a few minutes upon awakening), hypnagogic (falling asleep) hallucinations, insomnia, and motor parasomnias. Normal individuals pass through approximately 90 minutes of nonrapid eye movement (NREM) sleep (phases I to IV consecutively) before entering REM sleep. NREM sleep is a peaceful state of relaxation (low respiratory rate, muscle tone, BP) whereas REM sleep is characterized by physiologic and brain activity similar to wakefulness. Multiple Sleep Latency Tests (MSLTs) have demonstrated that patients with narcolepsy enter immediately into REM sleep from the waking state.

CASE CONTINUED

VS: 98.6°F BP 120/90 HR 76 RR16. Weight: 212 lbs Height: 5 ft 10 in

PE: Gen: Obese, well-groomed man. HEENT: WNL. Lungs: CTA. COR: RRR no murmurs.

Abdomen: Soft, nontender, nondistended.

Neuro: MSE: Mood is "okay," affect is appropriate, no psychomotor slowing is present. MMSE is 30/30.

CN II–XII: Intact

Motor: Normal bulk, tone, and strength in all four extremities

Reflexes: 2+ throughout. Babinski signs are absent bilaterally.

Sensory: Intact to light touch, pinprick, vibration, and temperature throughout.

Coordination: No nystagmus, dimetria, tremor, myoclonus, or dysdiadochokinesis is present.

Gait: Normal stance and gait. No ataxia, intact tandem gait. No Romberg sign is present.

QUESTIONS

49-1. What work-up should be ordered?
  A. All-night polysomnogram
  B. Thyroid function tests
  C. Chest radiograph
  D. MSLT
  E. A, B, and C

49-2. Suppose the sleep study showed more than four episodes of apnea lasting over 15 seconds, accompanied by at least a 10% drop in SaO$_2$. Which of the following is an appropriate treatment at this time?
A. CPAP
B. Modafinil
C. Amphetamines
D. Uvulopalatopharyngoplasty

49-3. Long-term complications of obstructive sleep apnea include:
A. Pulmonary HTN
B. Left ventricular failure
C. Sudden unexplained death
D. All of the above
E. A and C

49-4. Which of the following has been implicated in the pathogenesis of narcolepsy?
A. Obesity
B. HLA-DR2
C. Orexin deficiency
D. Mental retardation
E. All of the above

 ANSWERS

49-1. E. His clinical presentation is highly suggestive of obstructive sleep apnea. He is a middle-aged man, obese, with chronic daytime sleepiness, and his examination reveals diastolic HTN. An all-night polysomnogram should be ordered to document episodes of apnea lasting more than 10 seconds and accompanied by at least a 3% to 4% drop in SaO$_2$ and to assess the efficacy of a trial of CPAP. If he showed no evidence of apnea the next appropriate study would be a MSLT used to diagnose narcolepsy. Because he already shows evidence of diastolic HTN a chest radiograph should be done. Given his history of fatigue and weight gain thyroid function tests are also appropriate.

49-2. A. CPAP is the only consistently effective therapy for obstructive sleep apnea (OSA). However, many patients tolerate it poorly because the masks interfere with their sleep. This patient has not had anatomic studies of his neck and throat so we do not know whether an uvulopalatopharyngoplasty is indicated. In appropriate patients this is sometimes an effective surgical treatment. Amphetamines may improve his daytime sleepiness but are poor long-term treatments for OSA. Modafinil is used in the treatment of narcolepsy.

49-3. E. Right ventricular failure can result from untreated OSA. Other complications include systemic HTN, cardiac arrhythmias, polycythemia from hypercapnia, hypoxia, pulmonary HTN, and sudden unexplained death.

49-4. C. The etiology of narcolepsy is quite mysterious. There is a well-known association with HLA-DR2 locus, leading many investigators to postulate an autoimmune etiology. The disease usually begins between the ages of 10 and 30 years although diagnosis is often delayed. It is characterized by excessive daytime sleepiness, sleep attacks brought on by excitement, sleep paralysis, cataplexy, and hypnagogic hallucinations. The patients are intellectually normal. Recently, decreased levels of the neurotransmitter Orexin have been implicated in the pathophysiology.

 ADDITIONAL SUGGESTED READING

Scammell TE. The neurobiology, diagnosis, and treatment of narcolepsy. Ann Neurol 2003;53:154.

Zeman A, Britton T, Douglas N, et al. Narcolepsy and excessive daytime sleepiness. BMJ 2004;329:724.

Sleep Problems in Childhood

ID/CC: 5$^1/_2$-year-old girl who wakes up at night.

HPI: PN is a 5$^1/_2$-year-old girl who is brought to her pediatrician with the complaint of sleeping difficulty. As an infant she began sleeping through the night at 7 months of age. But for the past 2 weeks she wakes up in the middle of the night screaming, eyes open, and appears terrified. Despite best efforts, she cannot be consoled. Her parents are not even sure whether she was aware of what was happening. After crying inconsolably for several minutes, she stops and goes back to sleep. Upon waking up in the morning, she has no recollection of anything from the previous night. The first time it happened, her parents thought she was having a bad dream, but the frequent occurrence (almost every night) is concerning them.

Developmentally the child has met her milestones on time.

PMHx: Born at term, uneventful pregnancy and labor. History of bronchiolitis at 15 months of age, two episodes of wheezing with respiratory illnesses.

Meds: Albuterol MDI as needed

All: Erythromycin

FHx: 2-year-old brother with a history of crying spells (different from these)

SHx: Lives with parents and brother, attends a prekindergarten program.

VS: Temp 99°F, BP 90/54, HR 90, RR 22

PE: Gen: no dysmorphic features CV: normal heart sounds. Lungs: clear, no organomegaly. Skin, extremities, spine: normal.

Neuro: Alert, normal speech for age. Cranial nerve examination, motor examination: normal. Normal reflexes, coordination, and gait.

THOUGHT QUESTION

■ What is the differential diagnosis?

The major categories in the differential diagnosis of such paroxysmal events are seizures versus nonepileptic events. Among the paroxysmal nonepileptic disorders that occur in sleep the following should be considered:

Nightmares: These usually occur several hours after the child has fallen asleep (rapid eye movement [REM] sleep). The child may be restless, agitated during the episode, but it is unusual for the child to be inconsolably screaming. The child can often recall the dream (or at least parts of it).

Night terrors (pavor nocturnus): Common in children 4 to 10 years of age. These occur a few hours after going to sleep (non-REM [NREM] sleep). The child screams inconsolably, usually sits up. Eyes are open, but the child does not respond to people around her. The episodes last for 5 to 15 minutes, after which the child goes back to sleep, and has no recollection of the event the next morning.

Sleepwalking: As the name suggests, the child gets up a few hours after going to sleep and walks around, apparently in a trance. Eyes are open, mumbling speech (nonpurposeful) may be present. The child can be directed back into bed sometimes. There is no recollection of the event the next morning.

Seizures: Complex partial seizures may occur at night, and are usually associated with automatisms (semi- or nonpurposeful movements) other than walking. They tend to be brief, although abnormal, even wandering behavior may occur in the postictal state. Seizures of frontal lobe origin may have bizarre and complex behaviors and can be nocturnal, but tend to be brief (<40 seconds) in duration.

The distinction between a seizure and nonepileptic events coming out of sleep is usually clinical. In this case, the description of the event is classic for night terrors. A work-up is not needed, but if the diagnosis is in doubt, EEG studies (outpatient or video-EEG monitoring) may be used.

CASE CONTINUED

When further questioned, the child's parents describe her brother's crying spells as occurring when upset. He would cry inconsolably when upset, turn blue, and stop breathing. These spells were evaluated and deemed to be "benign." The spells stopped on their own a few months after they had begun.

THOUGHT QUESTION

■ What are the patient's brother's spells called?

The brother's spells are a typical example of breath-holding spells (BHS). These too can be mistaken for seizures, particularly as some BHS terminate with loss of consciousness. Diagnosis is on a clinical basis. EEG is normal.

QUESTIONS

50-1. BHS are most common at what age?
   A. 15 months
   B. 36 months
   C. 4 years
   D. 6 years

50-2. BHS are classified as:
   A. Simple and complex
   B. Cyanotic and pallid
   C. Either
   D. Neither

50-3. Night terrors may be accompanied by:
   A. Sleep walking
   B. Sleep apnea
   C. Nightmares
   D. All of the above

50-4. The natural history of night terrors is:
A. Higher incidence of epilepsy
B. Spontaneous remission
C. Resolution with pharmacologic treatment
D. School and behavior problems

 ANSWERS

50-1. A. BHS are common between the ages of 6 and 18 months. They usually occur in the setting of prolonged crying. The child cries relentlessly and then holds his breath. BHS may be accompanied by cyanosis, apnea, loss of muscle tone, pallor, and bradycardia. The episode is usually brief, lasting less than 1 minute. There tends to be a positive family history of BHS. These children are neurologically normal. BHS remit spontaneously by 6 years of age. No treatment is necessary. Where the diagnosis is in doubt (question of seizures), an EEG may be obtained, which is normal.

50-2. B. BHS are classified as cyanotic or pallid, depending on clinical signs of cyanosis or pallor during the event. The classification is purely descriptive, and the natural history and prognosis is the same for both types.

50-3. A. Night terrors may be accompanied by sleep walking. Both parasomnias occur out of NREM sleep.

50-4. B. Night terrors, while frightening for onlookers, are a benign condition. The child is neurologically normal. Once the diagnosis is established, reassurance is the only treatment required. In cases where the episodes are frequent or prolonged, treatment with a benzodiazepine at bedtime is useful. Night terrors remit spontaneously over time.

 ADDITIONAL SUGGESTED READING

Kupfer DJ, Reynolds CF. Current Concepts: management of insomnia. N Engl J Med 1997;336:341–346.

Difficulty Speaking in an Adult

ID/CC: 68-year-old man with difficulty speaking

HPI: AP is a 68-year-old right-handed man who presented to the ED with trouble speaking. His symptoms began on the morning of the day of presentation. When the patient woke up, he had difficulty expressing himself to his wife, difficulty telling her what he wanted to eat for breakfast. His wife said that his speech sounded unclear, like he was fumbling for words. His sentences were short and speech lacked fluency. His right arm was weak. His primary care physician was contacted and the patient was advised to go to the ED.

PMHx: HTN, hypothyroidism, history of a "small" stroke 5 years prior with left arm and right face weakness, from which he had made a complete recovery.

Meds: Atenolol, aspirin 81 mg per day

All: None

SHx: Quit drinking 10 years ago. Used to smoke 1 PPD, cut down after his earlier stroke, and now smokes a cigarette occasionally.

FHx: HTN and ischemic heart disease in his father, who died at age 74 of a myocardial infarction

VS: Afebrile, BP 165/95 HR 68 RR 18

PE: Gen: normal

Neuro: Mental status: Alert

Speech: Unable to name common objects like watch, shoe. Speech nonfluent and halting. Unable to repeat a sentence or phrase

CN exam: UMN pattern right facial weakness

Motor: Pronator drift on right upper extremity. Right UE strength 2/5, rest normal. Reflexes symmetric.

Sensory: Normal touch, pinprick, proprioception

THOUGHT QUESTION

■ What is this type of "difficulty speaking" called?

Acquired disorders of previously normal language function are called aphasias. Here the content of language is abnormal, and depending on the type of aphasia (Table 51-1), different aspects of language are affected. Speaking, reading, writing, comprehension, and repetition can be affected to varying degrees. Commonly language ability is tested at the bedside by asking the patient to name common objects, repeat words/phrases, read, and write.

Difficulty speaking because of dysfunction of muscles controlling articulation is called dysarthria. Here the content of speech, comprehension, reading, and writing are all normal, but spoken speech lacks clarity and is difficult to understand. Dysarthria can occur because of weakness of bulbar muscles, facial muscles, etc. (Table 51-1).

TABLE 51-1 Features of Aphasias

Aphasia	Fluency	Repetition	Comprehension
Broca	Nonfluent	Impaired	Relatively preserved
Wernicke	Fluent	Impaired	Impaired
Transcortical motor	Nonfluent	Intact	Intact
Transcortical sensory	Fluent	Intact	Intact
Conduction	Fluent	Impaired	Intact
Global	Nonfluent	Impaired	Impaired

CASE CONTINUED

Labs: CBC, chemistries: WNL. ECG: WNL.

Imaging: MRI scan of the brain shows two ischemic lesions: one in the left hemisphere, near the Sylvian fissure and a second in a different location (Fig. 51-1).

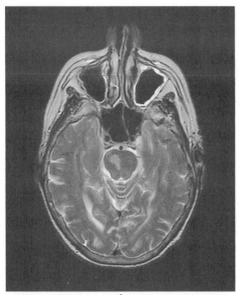

A

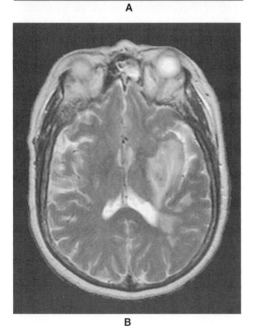

B

FIGURE 51-1
Axial images of MRI scan of the brain showing the patient's recent and remote strokes. (*Image courtesy of Dr. Ross Goldstein, Stanford University Medical Center, Stanford, California.*)

THOUGHT QUESTION

- Which lesion corresponds to the patient's present symptoms?

Of the two lesions, the lesion near the left Sylvian fissure is in an area supplied by the middle cerebral artery. This area encompasses speech centers such as the Broca (motor) and Wernicke (sensory) areas. The middle cerebral artery also supplies the region controlling the face and upper extremity. Anterior lesions will produce a motor aphasia and a prominent hemiparesis with predominant face and arm involvement. More posterior lesions will produce a sensory aphasia. The hemiparesis will be less prominent, and at times not be part of the symptoms and signs.

This lesion corresponds to the patient's present stroke.

The second lesion corresponds to the patient's old stroke.

QUESTIONS

51-1. Aphasia or other focal neurologic signs from which the patient recovers in 24 hours is called a:
   A. TIA
   B. Stroke
   C. Embolus
   D. Thrombus

51-2. Risk factors for stroke in this patient include all but which of the following?
   A. HTN
   B. Smoking
   C. Hypothyroidism
   D. Diabetes mellitus

51-3. Where was the patient's old stroke?
   A. Left internal capsule
   B. Right internal capsule
   C. Right pons
   D. Left pons

51-4. Medications used in the prevention of stroke include the following except:

    A. Aspirin

    B. Ibuprofen

    C. Clopidogrel

    D. Dipyridamole

 ANSWERS

51-1. A. The term TIA refers to focal neurologic symptoms that resolve in less than 24 hours. Focal neurologic symptoms that persist beyond 24 hours constitute the clinical entity of stroke or CVA. Thrombus and embolus are terms used to describe occlusion of blood vessels: thrombus is a clot that forms at the site of obstruction/occlusion of the blood vessel, embolus is a piece of clot that breaks off from its proximal source and occludes a distal vessel.

51-2. C. HTN, diabetes mellitus, and smoking are all recognized risk factors for cerebrovascular disease. Table 51-2 summarizes risk factors for stroke.

TABLE 51-2   Common Risk Factors for Stroke

Modifiable Factors
HTN
Diabetes mellitus
Hyperlipidemia
Ischemic heart disease
Atrial fibrillation
Smoking
Obesity
Oral contraceptives
Excessive alcohol use
Prior history of stroke
Nonmodifiable factors
Age
Male gender
Family history of stroke
Race (higher incidence in Asians, African-Americans)

51-3. C. The patient's previous stroke (hemiparesis with contralateral facial weakness) is because of a lesion in the brainstem contralateral to the extremity weakness. The facial weakness will be a LMN pattern facial weakness. The lesion that produces such a pattern of weakness is in the right pons.

51-4. B. Aspirin, clopidogrel and dipyridamole are used in stroke prevention. All three drugs inhibit platelet aggregation.

 ADDITIONAL SUGGESTED READING

Neary D, Snowden JS, Gustafson L, et al. Frontotemporal lobar degeneration: a consensus on clinical diagnostic criteria. Neurology 1998;51:1546.

IX

Patients Who Present with Vertigo, Diplopia, and Facial Weakness

Vomiting, Vertigo, and Ataxia

 CC: 65-year-old Vietnamese man presents with sudden onset of nausea, vomiting, vertigo, and ataxia.

HPI: One hour ago, IS was working in his garden with his wife when he suddenly became dizzy and nauseous and began vomiting. He was unable to walk to his house because of severe unsteadiness and was immediately brought to the hospital via ambulance. The vertigo and vomiting are somewhat relieved when lying down. On neurologic review of systems he also complains of numbness on the left side of his face and his wife notes a change in his voice. Mr. S denies any similar previous events.

PMHx: HTN

PSHx: None

Meds: Metoprolol

All: NKDA

SHx: Smoker, 1 PPD for 50 years

FHx: Heart disease and diabetes

Neuro Hx: None

THOUGHT QUESTIONS

- What is the most likely diagnosis and what are his risk factors?
- What are the different possible etiologies of this type of stroke?

283

The most likely diagnosis is a stroke. Although nausea, vomiting, vertigo, and mild ataxia are also symptoms of acute labyrinthitis, the ataxia does not prevent ambulation as it does in this patient. Additionally, the abruptness of the onset of symptoms, facial numbness, and his multiple stroke risk factors strongly argue against an inner ear disturbance. His risk factors for a stroke include his age, sex, ethnicity, heavy smoking history, and HTN. People of Asian and African descent are more likely to have intracranial stenoses and particularly Asians have a higher incidence of posterior circulation strokes as compared with whites.

The general differential diagnoses for causes of such a stroke include: (1) local thrombotic occlusion because of intracranial atherosclerosis; (2) embolic occlusion either from an intracardiac thrombus or vegetation or, less likely in this case, from an artery-to-artery embolus; (3) intracranial posterior fossa hemorrhage (cerebellum or pons), most often because of uncontrolled HTN or hemorrhagic conversion of a large ischemic infarct; (4) lacunar infarct because of degeneration (occlusion and/or rupture) of the cerebral microcirculation (this is very common in diabetics and patients with longstanding HTN); and (5) inflammatory involvement of the posterior circulation because of a primary or secondary CNS vasculitis.

CASE CONTINUED

VS: Temp 98.6°F BP 180/90 HR 76 RR 16

PE: Gen: No carotid bruits or cardiac murmur is auscultated.

Neuro: MMSE: Patient is coherent and oriented. He vomits several times during the exam.

Cranial nerves: Visual fields are full. Funduscopic exam is normal. The left pupil is slightly smaller than the right but responds to light and accommodation. Mild left-sided ptosis is present. There is decreased sensation to temperature and pinprick over the left side of the face. Extraocular movements are intact. Facial strength is symmetrical bilaterally. Left soft palate does not elevate and gag reflex is diminished. Voice is hoarse. Bedside swallow testing is markedly abnormal. Tongue is midline. Sternocleidomastoid strength is intact bilaterally.

Motor: Strength, bulk, and tone are intact bilaterally.

Reflexes: 2+ throughout. Babinski signs present bilaterally.

Sensory: Diminished pain and temperature sensation of the right trunk, arm, and leg. Light touch and vibration are intact throughout.

Coordination: Severe dysmetria in the left arm and leg. Right side is intact. No tremor is noted. Severe, symmetrical nystagmus with lateral gaze to the left and right.

Gait: Wide based, severe ataxia. Patient unable to ambulate.

 CASE CONTINUED

You can see from his PE that his left V, IX, and X cranial nerves are affected.

The diminished left-sided facial sensation is because of damage to the nucleus of the trigeminal nerve (V). The asymmetry in the palate is because of damage of the left glossopharyngeal nerve (IX) and the dysphagia is because of damage of both the IX and X (vagus) cranial nerves. The hypoglossal nerve (XII) is unaffected as demonstrated by normal tongue movements. His asymmetric pupil, which responds to light and accommodation along with the ptosis, is a classic description of a Horner's syndrome. A Horner's syndrome results from damage to the pre- or postganglionic sympathetic fibers of the superior cervical ganglion. In this case, it is because of damage of the preganglionic fibers that traverse the brainstem. The optic and oculomotor cranial nerves are not affected.

 QUESTIONS

52-1. Where does his lesion localize to?
   A. Left lateral pons
   B. Left lateral medulla
   C. Right lateral medulla
   D. Right lateral medulla and inferior cerebellar peduncle
   E. Left lateral medulla and inferior cerebellar peduncle

52-2. Occlusion of which artery can cause this syndrome?
   A. Posterior inferior cerebellar artery
   B. Superior cerebellar artery
   C. Vertebral artery
   D. A and C
   E. None of the above

52-3. The CT scan shows no evidence of a posterior fossa hemorrhage. What is the most appropriate treatment at this time?
   A. IV recombinant tissue plasminogen activator
   B. IV heparin
   C. Aspirin
   D. Supportive care
   E. Intra-arterial recombinant tissue plasminogen activator

52-4. Suppose the patient's CT scan showed a large cerebellar hemorrhage and the patient was rapidly losing consciousness. What emergent treatment options should be presented to the family at that time?
   A. IV mannitol, intubation, and hyperventilation
   B. Surgical decompression of the posterior fossa (craniotomy)
   C. Barbiturate coma
   D. A and B

ANSWERS

52-1. E. This is a classic description of a lateral medullary syndrome (Wallenberg's syndrome), which results from damage to the lateral medulla and the inferior cerebellar peduncle. The combination of an ipsilateral Horner's syndrome, loss of pain and temperature in the ipsilateral face (descending tract of the fifth nerve) and contralateral body (spinothalamic tract), damage to the lower vestibular nuclei (nausea, vomiting, nystagmus, and vertigo) and damage to the ninth and tenth cranial nerves (dysphagia and hoarseness) are all because of infarction of the lateral medulla. The ipsilateral ataxia (which may or may not be accompanied by diminished reflexes) results from damage to the inferior cerebellar peduncle.

52-2. D. Blood supply to the lateral medulla is variable and infarction of this territory can be because of either occlusion of the posterior inferior cerebellar artery or the parent vertebral artery.

52-3. A. This patient meets the criteria for treatment with IV recombinant tissue-type plasminogen activator (rt-PA) and therefore should be offered this. He arrived at the hospital shortly after his stroke and has neither unstable HTN, evidence of extensive infarction, or blood on his CT scan or other medical conditions to preclude its use. The sooner this medication is given (despite the 3-hour window) the more likely it is to not induce serious complications (hemorrhage); thus timeliness is extremely important. Intra-arterial thrombolytic agents have been given in the setting of vertebrobasilar occlusions up to 24 hours after the onset of symptoms; however, the efficacy and safety of this route of administration has yet to be demonstrated.

52-4. D. Hemorrhage of the cerebellum is a life-threatening condition because it often results in severe edema and compression of the brainstem, as indicated in this question by the loss of consciousness. Emergent treatment options that sometimes prove effective are the use of an anti-edema agent such as IV mannitol, hyperventilation to achieve hypercapnia also aimed at decreasing edema, and, in some cases, surgical decompression of the posterior fossa. Despite these treatments, however, the prognosis remains poor. Inducing coma with barbiturates (typically a short-acting agent such as thiopental) is often considered as a last resort in the treatment of increased intracranial pressure following severe head injury based largely on case series and observational studies. However, it has never been shown to be useful in the setting of increased intracranial pressure following stroke and is contraindicated because of the substantial risk of systemic hypotension with the use of barbiturates, which in case series reports has worsened stroke outcomes.

 ADDITIONAL SUGGESTED READING

Imai T, Ito M, Takeda N, et al. Natural course of the remission of vertigo in patients with benign paroxysmal positional vertigo. Neurology 2005;64:920.

Neuhauser H, Leopold M, von Brevern M, et al. The interrelations of migraine, vertigo, and migrainous vertigo. Neurology 2001;56:436.

Dizziness, Vomiting, and Imbalance

ID/CC: 38-year-old man presents with acute onset of dizziness, nausea, vomiting, and imbalance.

HPI: NS was in his usual state of good health until yesterday when he noticed a sensation of fullness in his ear, mild dizziness, and unsteadiness while getting ready for bed. That night while rolling over in bed he was aroused to complete alertness by severe dizziness, nausea, and vomiting. He describes the dizziness as a room-spinning sensation, counter-clockwise, that is significantly worsened with any head movement. The dizziness is improved with lying flat but does not resolve. He has been unable to hold down any food or liquids because each time he sits upright for more than a few minutes he begins vomiting. He has been able to ambulate around his house mostly by leaning on walls. His wife drove him to the emergency room. He denies any facial numbness, diplopia, or headache. He has never had a similar episode.

PMHx: None

PSHx: Arthroscopic knee surgery 10 years prior

Meds: None

All: NKDA

SHx: Insurance salesman. Married with 3 children. Non-smoker, drinks 1 beer per day.

FHx: Maternal: migraine headaches; paternal: HTN, heart disease

Neuro Hx: Suffers from classic migraine headaches with a visual aura since childhood

THOUGHT QUESTIONS

▪ Where could his lesion localize?

▪ List a broad differential diagnosis for vertigo and dizziness.

The first step in these cases is to clarify what the patient means by "dizziness." The main distinction to make is between light-headedness and vertigo. Key questions include whether they experience a sensation of movement where there is none (spinning, side-to-side, etc.), whether they feel as though they will pass out, and whether the sensation comes on in relation to position (lying, sitting, standing) or movement (turning, sitting up, reaching over their head).

Vertigo and dizziness can be caused by: (1) damage to the peripheral vestibular end organs (semicircular canals, utricle, and saccule) or the vestibular portion of the eighth nerve; (2) CNS disease affecting the vestibular nuclei in the brainstem or the central vestibular neural pathways mostly located in the cerebellum; and (3) systemic causes.

The differential diagnosis for an acute attack of vertigo, nausea, vomiting, and imbalance by categories are as follows: (1) peripheral causes include a peripheral vestibulopathy (labyrinthitis or neuronitis), benign positional vertigo, Ménière's disease, vestibulotoxic drug ingestion (gentamicin is a common cause) and local ENT abnormalities (bacterial infection, otosclerosis, perilymph fistula); (2) central causes include demyelinating disease (multiple sclerosis, paraneoplastic syndrome), brainstem ischemia or infarction, cerebellopontine angle tumors (acoustic neuroma, metastatic tumor, meningioma), brainstem arteriovenous malformation (AVM) or tumor, cerebellar lesion (tumor or hematoma), and spinocerebellar degeneration; (3) systemic causes—drugs (antihypertensives, alcohol, tranquilizers, hypnotics, analgesics, and anticonvulsants), hypotension and presyncope, hematologic disorders (anemia, polycythemia and dysproteinemia), diabetes, hypothyroidism, meningitis, vasculitis, and granulomatous disease.

Peripheral and systemic causes of vertigo are more common than central causes.

CASE CONTINUED

VS: Temp 98.6°F BP 140/80 HR 86 RR 16

PE: Gen: HEENT: Tympanic membranes clear. No thyromegaly. Neck is supple.

COR: RRR no murmurs

Neuro: MSE: Patient is alert and oriented times 4. Speech is clear and coherent. Answers questions appropriately. Clearly uncomfortable during the parts of the exam that require sitting up or ambulating. Vomits once during the course of the exam.

CNS: Visual fields are full, PERRLA, extra-ocular movement intact (EOMI). Unable to visualize fundi because of nystagmus. Facial strength and sensation are intact. Hearing is intact bilaterally. Uvula and tongue are midline. Gag reflex is present. Bedside swallow evaluation is normal. Sternocleidomastoid strength is equal bilaterally.

Motor: Normal bulk, tone, and strength in all four extremities

Reflexes: 2+ throughout. Babinski signs absent bilaterally.

Sensory: Intact to light touch, pinprick, vibration, and temperature in all four extremities

Coordination: Spontaneous and gaze-evoked horizontal nystagmus is present. The fast phase of the nystagmus is toward the right. The nystagmus increases in intensity with right lateral gaze. Nystagmus disappears during straightforward gaze when the patient is lying down. On finger-to-nose testing patient misses your finger several times, past-pointing to the right. The movements are smooth with no tremor or jerking motions present.

Gait: Stance is normal. With ambulation patient occasionally staggers to the right. Romberg sign is not testable because the patient becomes too dizzy and nauseous with standing.

QUESTIONS

53-1. Based on his history and PE, where does his lesion localize?
A. Right cerebellum
B. Left cerebellum
C. Right peripheral vestibular organ
D. Left peripheral vestibular organ

53-2. What work-up should be done?
A. Brain MRI
B. Electronystagmography
C. Caloric stimulation
D. Audiometry
E. None of the above

53-3. Suppose the episode improves with special head positioning maneuvers. What is the most likely diagnosis?
A. Vestibular neuronitis
B. Cerebello-pontine angle tumor
C. Benign paroxysmal positional vertigo
D. Ménière's disease

53-4. All of his symptoms resolve over several weeks. Six months later he comes to your office with a very similar attack lasting several hours and leaving him feeling "off balance," only this time the vertigo came on so suddenly he fell to the ground. What work-up should be ordered?
A. Brain MRI
B. Audiometry testing and referral to ENT specialist
C. Moving platform posturography test
D. EEG

ANSWERS

53-1. D. This is a classic description of an acute left vestibular neuronitis (inflammation, often viral, of the vestibular nerve). The acute phase of the attack usually lasts 5 to 7 days and full recovery often takes weeks. The onset is characterized by severe vertigo and ataxia, with or without N&V. Methylprednisolone has been shown to improve symptoms in the acute phase. During the recovery phase the patients often complain of a persistent sensation of imbalance.

In peripheral vestibular disease the nystagmus is horizontal or rotary and extinguishes with fixation in a neutral position. The nystagmus is worse with lateral gaze away from the lesion and the fast phase of the nystagmus occurs opposite the side of the lesion. In central causes of vertigo the nystagmus is often multidirectional and does not extinguish. The ataxia is a result of the imbalance of vestibular input and not because of cerebellar or spinal cord disease. Clinically, the patients can walk, albeit with difficulty, but are usually limited by the vertigo and nausea. Past-pointing opposite the side of the lesion on finger-to-nose testing is a common finding during the acute phase. A cerebellar lesion would produce not only past-pointing but also lack of smoothness of the movement (i.e., dysmetria).

53-2. E. All of the clinical information needed to make a diagnosis and to localize the lesion has been given in the H&P. If there were some question about which side the lesion localized to or the nature of the nystagmus (horizontal, rotational, or multidirectional) electronystagmography would be useful. Caloric stimulation could help localize the lesion as well; however, in conscious patients it usually induces severe vertigo and nausea and for that reason is now usually reserved for severely encephalopathic or comatose patients. The patient has no auditory abnormalities and nothing on examination to point toward a central etiology, thus auditory testing or brain MRI are not necessary at this time.

53-3. C. Vestibular neuronitis (vestibular neuritis, labyrinthitis) and benign paroxysmal positional vertigo (BPPV) are the most common causes of peripheral vertigo. Vestibular neuronitis does not usually improve with head maneuvers. BPPV is characterized by brief episodes (seconds to minutes) of vertigo and nystagmus triggered by head movement in any direction and resolving with maintaining the new head position. The attacks are recurrent and are thought to be caused by debris in the semicircular canals leading to irritation. The nystagmus on examination lessens (fatigues) with repeated provocative maneuvers. The treatment for BPPV is Eply maneuvers (positioning the head in various ways to try to facilitate removal of debris from the affected canal) and supportive care (bed rest, fluids, deep vein thrombosis [DVT] prophylaxis) during the acute phase and vestibular exercises during the recovery phase. To lessen the vertigo during the acute phase, anticholinergic drugs (meclizine, transdermal scopolamine), antihistamines, and sympathomimetic agents (amphetamines or ephedrine) are often prescribed, as are antiemetics and tranquilizers to make the patient more comfortable.

53-4. B. The differential diagnosis for recurrent attacks of vertigo and ataxia include recurrent vestibular neuronitis, BPPV, Ménière's disease, basilar migraines, complex partial seizures, vertebrobasilar TIAs, and familial periodic ataxia. In this patient the clue to the diagnosis is the severity of onset of the attack (falling to the ground), the preceding sensation of fullness in his ear, and his age. Ménière's disease is a rare condition caused by an increase in volume of endolymphatic fluid, resulting in distension of the semicircular canals. Clinically, it is characterized by recurrent attacks of severe vertigo usually lasting hours, some of which are so severe they cause the patient to fall to the ground. The vertigo is usually preceded by a sensation of fullness, decreased hearing and tinnitus in one ear. A chronic sense of imbalance can persist between episodes. It usually begins in the third and fourth decades of life. During an episode, audiometry testing often reveals a low-tone sensorineural hearing loss that can resolve between attacks. With repeated attacks the hearing loss often becomes progressive and permanent. Treatment of an acute attack is similar to that of an attack of vestibular neuronitis. Thiazide or acetazolamide diuretics and a low-sodium diet are also often recommended, although their efficacy is not clear. A variety of surgical options are available for treatment of intractable disease to improve and prevent hearing loss. Although the diagnosis is most likely Ménière's disease, the patient should also be referred to ENT specialist to rule out other rare but often surgically treatable abnormalities of the inner ear (otosclerosis or labyrinth fistula) that can result in recurrent attacks of vertigo.

 ADDITIONAL SUGGESTED READING

Baloh RW. Clinical practice: vestibular neuritis. N Engl J Med 2003;348:1027.

Furman JM, Hain TC. "Do try this at home": self-treatment of BPPV. Neurology 2004;63:8.

Tusa RJ. Vertigo. Neurol Clin 2001;19:23.

Diplopia

ID/CC: 29-year-old woman complains of double vision.

HPI: BD first noticed the double vision three days ago at which time it was intermittent. It has steadily worsened since then and is now almost constant. She has started covering one eye in order to carry out her household tasks without bumping into things. She denies any ocular pain or headaches. Over the last 3 months she has also experienced intermittent tingling and numbness in her hands, diagnosed as postpartum carpal tunnel syndrome by her OB. She is 6 months postpartum. The remainder of her neurologic review of systems is negative except for fatigue since delivery. She also denies any fevers, chills, night sweats, or episodes of loss of consciousness or confusion.

PMHx: None

PSHx: None

Meds: Ibuprofen and Dulcolax

All: NKDA

SHx: Engineer, married with two children

FHx: Thyroid disease

Neuro Hx: 10 years ago she experienced numbness in her feet following a long day of skiing. The numbness resolved over the next month.

THOUGHT QUESTIONS

- Where could her lesion(s) localize? (at least three possibilities)
- What signs will you look for on examination to aid in localization?

■ Describe the expected abnormal eye movements seen in a right isolated third, fourth, or sixth nerve palsy.

Binocular diplopia can result from (1) weakness of the extraocular muscles, often because of neuromuscular disease or entrapment of extraocular muscles following orbital fracture; (2) a disease process affecting any of the cranial nerves that control eye movements (III, IV, VI) or their nuclei, which includes a broad list including diabetes, cavernous sinus thrombosis, meningioma, intracranial aneurysm, thyrotoxicosis, and stroke; and (3) lesions of the medial longitudinal fasciculus (MLF). Symmetrical hand paresthesias can result from disease processes affecting the peripheral nerves (frequently systemic diseases), entrapment syndrome, or cervical cord disease.

To aid in localization important things to look for on examination are: (1) ptosis, facial weakness, and LMN signs (neuromuscular disease); (2) proptosis, redness and swelling of the upper face and orbit, visual acuity, pupillary responses to light (for disease processes compressing cranial nerves III, IV, or VI); (3) position of the pupils in straightforward gaze, symmetry of eye movements and nystagmus (determine which cranial nerve or whether the MLF is affected); (4) distribution of the paresthesias and LMN signs in hands (peripheral neuropathy or entrapment syndrome; and (5) a sensory level, posterior column signs (vibration and joint position sense) and UMN signs (for cervical cord disease) (Fig. 54-1).

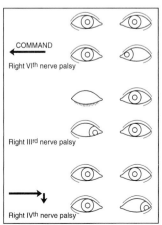

FIGURE 54-1 Isolated right cranial nerve palsies. (*Illustration by Electronic Illustrators Group.*)

CASE CONTINUED

VS: Temp 98.6°F BP 110/70 HR 76 RR 16

PE: Gen: no facial swelling or redness, no proptosis, no thyromegaly

Neuro: CN II: PERRLA, visual acuity 20/20 OU. Eye movements (CN III, IV, VI): Eyes are midline in forward gaze. Patient reports diplopia is worse on extreme lateral gaze in both directions. Unable to adduct either eye with marked nystagmus in the abducting eye; when eyes are tested separately, adduction improves. Weakness of convergence in both eyes. CN V, VII–XII: intact.

Motor: Normal bulk, tone, and strength in the bilateral upper and lower extremities; no fatiguing weakness; normal neck flexion strength, no ptosis

Reflexes: 2+ throughout. Babinski signs present bilaterally.

Sensory: Diminished to light touch, pain, and vibration bilateral hands to the wrist; C8 sensory level

Coordination: Positive Romberg, no tremor, or dysmetria

Gait: No ataxia

QUESTIONS

54-1. How would you describe her eye movement abnormalities?
   A. Bilateral cranial nerve IV palsies
   B. Symmetrical internuclear ophthalmoplegia
   C. Bilateral partial cranial nerve VI palsies
   D. Bilateral partial cranial nerve III palsies

54-2. What other lesion(s) does she have?
   A. Cervical cord
   B. Cerebellar
   C. Peripheral nerve
   D. Cervical cord and cerebellar

54-3. What is the most likely diagnosis?
   A. Lyme's disease
   B. Multiple sclerosis
   C. Diabetes
   D. Vitamin B12 deficiency

54-4. Her brain and cervical cord MRI reveal four hyperintense lesions on T2-weighted images, of which enhances with gadolinium on T1-weighted sequences. Which of the following would be an appropriate next step?

    A. Treat with interferon-β-1a
    B. Treat with interferon-β-1b
    C. Treat with copolymer-1
    D. Treat with corticosteroids
    E. Perform a LP, then start treatment
    F. All of the above

ANSWERS

54-1. B. This is a classic description of a symmetrical internuclear ophthalmoplegia (INO). Her INO is because of symmetrical lesions of the MLF. The MLF traverses the pons and midbrain and is important in coordinating conjugate lateral eye movements performed by cranial nerves III and VI. Cranial nerve VI lesions would result in abnormalities of abduction. Cranial nerve IV palsies would result in the down- and outward deviation of the outward looking eye on lateral gaze. While partial III palsies would result in abnormal adduction of each eye, it does not improve when the eyes are tested separately and is usually accompanied by ptosis.

54-2. A. Her sensory level, posterior column sign (diminished vibration), and positive Romberg are all a reflection of a cervical cord lesion. While positive Romberg sign can also be caused by peripheral neuropathy, vestibular disease or cerebellar lesions, the remainder of her examination did not reveal any other cerebellar signs (dysmetria, tremor or ataxia). The distribution of her sensory deficits is not consistent with carpal tunnel syndrome or other peripheral nerve lesion.

54-3. B. Bilateral INO is virtually pathognomonic for multiple sclerosis (MS). Other rare but important causes of symmetrical INO are anticonvulsant toxicity and, in children, pontine gliomas. Unilateral INO is usually because of brainstem strokes. This patient has other typical features of MS including a cervical cord lesion, a history of paresthesias, onset of symptoms over several days, age, female gender, and the occurrence of an attack in the postpartum period. The episode of leg numbness several years ago, which the patient attributed to skiing, most likely was her first attack of the disease. A typical symptom of MS, not mentioned in this case, is the brief (usually minutes to hours) return of neurologic deficits with increased body temperature (most often during exercise, hot showers, and hot summers) that resolve once the patient's body temperature returns to normal. This heat sensitivity, also known as Uhthoff phenomenon, does not reflect new disease activity.

MS is an inflammatory demyelinating disease of the CNS. Like rheumatoid arthritis, it is a female-predominating T-cell mediated autoimmune disease that typically improves during pregnancy and flares in the postpartum period. The prevalence of MS worldwide varies greatly and a higher frequency is found in countries farthest north of the equator with the exception of Greenland. In North America the prevalence is 60 in 100,000 and appears to be increasing. While MS has been linked in small series to many potential infectious agents (mumps, measles, Epstein-Barr virus, herpes virus, hepatitis B, and *Chlamydia pneumoniae*) a causal relationship in larger patient series continuously fails to be shown. Additionally, the infectious agents are all ubiquitous and an adequate explanation of how they may lead to MS in only a few infected individuals has not been shown. A genetic component modulating susceptibility to MS seems likely and genetic linkage studies have identified HLA DR2 as a risk factor in white patients with sporadic MS. Fifteen percent to 20% of MS patients have an affected relative (first, second, and third degree) with MS and the risk of developing MS in first-degree relatives of affected individuals is 3% to 5%. Extensive genetic studies of familial MS, thus far, have failed to demonstrate any one specific gene defect. Thus, it appears most likely that several genes influence the susceptibility to MS.

54-4. F. This woman meets all of the criteria for clinically and laboratory-supported definite MS with a relapsing-remitting course (relapsing-remitting multiple sclerosis [RRMS]). She has had two attacks separated in time and an MRI scan that supports the diagnosis. There are three immunomodulatory treatments available in the United States that are effective in diminishing the relapse rate in RRMS: interferon-β-1a, interferon-β-1b and copolymer-1. Treatment with one of these three medications should be offered immediately to this patient. While treatment with corticosteroids (typically methylprednisolone IV 1 g a day for 3 to 5 days) may help speed her recovery from this exacerbation, it will not slow the progression of her disease. While a LP is not necessary to establish a diagnosis of MS in this patient, the presence of oligoclonal bands, increased IgG index, and no or minimal lymphocytic pleocytosis (15 cells/μL) are hallmarks of the disease and would make any other diseases that can mimic MS extremely unlikely. The presence of a lymphocytic pleocytosis over 50 cells/μL should prompt the investigation for other etiologies.

 ADDITIONAL SUGGESTED READING

Patel SV, Holmes JM, Hodge DO, et al. Diabetes and HTN in isolated sixth nerve palsy: a population-based study. Ophthalmology 2005;112:760.

Diplopia and Dysphagia

ID/CC: 37-year-old woman complains of double vision, fatigue, and difficulty swallowing.

HPI: Over the last 3 weeks MS has noticed worsening diplopia, particularly in the late afternoons. One week ago she was diagnosed with multiple sclerosis and prescribed an oral course of prednisone. Over the last 3 days she has developed intermittent weakness in her legs following long walks, difficulty swallowing, and worsening diplopia. She denies any numbness, nausea, vomiting, diarrhea, blurred vision, fever, or night sweats.

PMHx:	None
PSHx:	None
Meds:	Prednisone 60 mg by mouth once a day
All:	NKDA
SHx:	Engineer, married with two children
FHx:	Thyroid disease
Neuro Hx:	None

THOUGHT QUESTIONS

- Where could her lesion(s) localize? (at least three possibilities)
- What signs will you look for on examination to aid in localization?
- Name three diseases that affect the neuromuscular junction and discuss clinical clues used to differentiate between them.

Diplopia, dysphagia, and paraparesis can result from disease processes affecting:

1. Multiple cranial and peripheral nerves
2. Neuromuscular junction
3. Alpha motor neurons in the anterior horn of the spinal cord and brainstem
4. CNS lesion(s) affecting midbrain (diplopia), brainstem (diplopia, dysphagia, and paraparesis) and/or spinal cord (paraparesis)

To aid in localization important signs to look for on examination are:

1. LMN signs (hyporeflexia, weakness, hypotonia, muscular atrophy, fasciculations)
2. UMN signs (hyperreflexia, excessive gag, spasticity, Babinski signs)
3. Fatiguing weakness (worsening muscle strength with repeated testing or prolonged contraction)
4. Sensory involvement (this would exclude alpha motor neuron disease or neuromuscular junction disorder)
5. Ptosis
6. Bulbar weakness

The three major diseases that affect the neuromuscular junction (NMJ) are MG, botulism, and LEMS. Of these MG is the most common NMJ disorder in the United States. The age of onset of MG has a bimodal peak and unequal sex distribution: women ages 20 to 35 years and men and women in their 60s and 70s. In young women the disease typically presents with variable ptosis, ocular weakness, and dysarthria, dysphagia, or weakness with chewing. Fifteen percent of all patients with MG have abnormalities limited to the extraocular and eyelid muscles only while the majority (85%) of MG patients have generalized weakness involving the limbs, diaphragm, and neck extensors. The weakness is characterized by diurnal variation of weakness (usually better in the morning and worse in the late afternoon) and increasing weakness with repeated use of the same muscle groups (fatiguing weakness).

Botulism is caused by ingestion of botulinum toxin or wound botulism (usually from penetrating wounds or IV drug abuse). The toxin inhibits presynaptic release of acetylcholine (Ach), causing permanent damage to cholinergic nerve terminals. Recovery is by sprouting of new fibers and requires a prolonged period of hospitalization. The onset of disease is much more rapid than in MG or LEMS. Following ingestion or infection the patient is asymptomatic for 8 to 36 hours and then develops symptoms of muscarinic Ach transmission disruption first (nausea, diarrhea, blurred vision, sore throat and mouth), loss of pupillary reactions, an important early diagnostic clue, followed by weakness. Unlike MG and LEMS, the weakness follows a characteristic descending pattern with ophthalmoparesis and bulbar symptoms (dysphagia) preceding limb weakness.

LEMS is caused by antibodies directed against voltage gated calcium channels in the presynaptic terminal resulting in decreased Ach release and subsequently decreased stimulation of both nicotinic and muscarinic Ach receptors although symptoms from muscarinic disruption are much less common. Weakness is predominantly proximal, affecting the legs more than the arms and improves with repeated use. Areflexia is common. Sixty percent of patients with LEMS have an underlying tumor (most commonly small-cell lung cancer) and 75% of these patients present with LEMS prior to the diagnosis of the cancer.

 CASE CONTINUED

VS: Temp 98.6°F BP 110/70 HR 76 RR 24

PE: Gen: No thyromegaly. No rashes.

Neuro: CN II: PERRLA. CN III, IV, VI mild asymmetric ptosis bilaterally, variable eye movement abnormalities with repeated testing. CN V: facial sensation intact. CN VII: mild bifacial weakness with cheeks puffed, able to raise eyebrows. CN VIII: hearing intact. CN IX, X, and XII: tongue and uvula midline. Palate elevates symmetrically. Diminished gag reflex. CN XI: intact sternocleidomastoid (SCM) strength bilaterally.

Motor: Normal strength, tone, and bulk of all muscle groups to direct testing. After prolonged neck flexion, arm and leg raise strength 4/5. No fasciculations.

Reflexes: 2+ throughout. No Babinski signs are present.

Sensory: Intact to light touch, pinprick, vibration, and joint position sense

Coordination: No tremor, dysmetria, nystagmus, or dysdiadochokinesis

Gait: Normal, no ataxia

QUESTIONS

55-1. Her lesion(s) localize to:
A. Peripheral nerves
B. NMJ
C. Alpha motor neuron disease
D. CNS

55-2. Which diagnostic tests should be ordered?
A. Edrophonium test
B. EMG with repeated stimulation
C. Vital capacity and arterial blood gas (ABG)
D. Brain and spinal cord MRI scan
E. All of the above

55-3. Suppose the result of her edrophonium test is positive. What additional work-up should be ordered?
A. Serum anti-acetylcholine receptor antibodies
B. Thyroid function tests
C. Chest CT
D. Serum anti-calcium channel antibodies
E. A, B, and C
F. All of the above

55-4. Which treatment course would you recommend?
A. Stop prednisone and start pyridostigmine as an outpatient
B. Admit patient, continue prednisone, and start pyridostigmine
C. Decrease the dose of prednisone and start pyridostigmine as an outpatient
D. Add pyridostigmine and send the patient home
E. Admit patient and perform a thymectomy

ANSWERS

55-1. B. The combination of fatiguing weakness, ptosis, variable eye movement abnormalities, preserved muscle stretch reflexes, hypoactive gag reflex, and absence of sensory involvement all point to a NMJ disorder. Although there are forms of subacute progressive peripheral polyneuropathies that do not affect sensory fibers, they would produce hyporeflexia. In the case of alpha motor neuron disease (poliomyelitis or ALS) one would expect to find hyporeflexia and fixed weakness to direct muscle group testing on exam not fatiguing weakness. She has no UMN signs to point to a diagnosis of multiple sclerosis or other CNS disease.

55-2. E. Her presentation is classic for MG. To perform the edrophonium test (or Tensilon test) edrophonium, an anticholinesterase, and saline control are administered intravenously and the patient is monitored for improvement of neuromuscular weakness by a blinded observer. The patient must also be monitored for hypotension and bradycardia as well and a crash cart with intubation material and atropine must be on hand. If they are not available do not perform this test! Obvious improvement in neuromuscular weakness following administration of Tensilon but not following saline is considered a positive test and strongly suggests a diagnosis of myasthenia gravis. To confirm the diagnosis of MG and EMG with repetitive stimulation should show a decremental response. NCV and MRI are not necessary. MG can lead to diaphragmatic weakness, particularly after the initiation of corticosteroid treatment, and she already exhibits bulbar symptoms and signs (dysphagia, bifacial weakness, and diminished gag) and has tachypnea. Bifacial weakness often prevents patients from forming a tight seal when forced vital capacity is tested and may therefore be inaccurate, thus an ABG should be done as well to rule out significant respiratory compromise.

55-3. E. MG is an autoimmune disease characterized by fluctuating, fatiguing weakness caused by blocking antibodies directed at the Ach receptor on the postsynaptic membrane in the neuromuscular junction. Over time, this results in simplification of the folding pattern in the postsynaptic membrane and an increased gap between the pre- and postsynaptic nerve terminals. Muscarinic receptors are not affected in MG. The antibody titers correlate directly with disease severity in most patients although 10% to 20% of patients have Ab negative MG. Hyperthyroidism is present in 3% to 8% of MG patients and exacerbates the condition. Seventy-five percent of MG patients have associated thymic abnormalities (thymic hyperplasia or thymoma) and may benefit from thymectomy. For this reason a chest CT scan should be performed on all newly diagnosed MG patients.

55-4. B. Newly diagnosed MG patients with evidence of generalized disease such as this patient (i.e., not confined to the extraocular muscles) are treated with oral pyridostigmine, an anticholinesterase, for symptomatic control and prednisone to control the underlying autoimmune process. Unlike in MS treatment, prednisone is started at a low dose, 15 to 20 mg/day, and increased slowly to 50 to 60 mg once a day because it can initially worsen MG symptoms as it did in this patient. Because she shows evidence of bulbar and respiratory compromise and is on high-dose prednisone she should be monitored closely and under no circumstances be sent home. While thymectomy may be a useful long-term treatment depending on the results of her chest CT, it is not the first-line treatment during a myasthenic crisis. Prior to discharge she should be counseled about the numerous medications that can precipitate a myasthenic crisis, encouraged to contact the MG foundation and to carry a list of these precipitants with her.

 ADDITIONAL SUGGESTED READING

Burns TM, Russell JA, LaChance DH, et al. Oculobulbar involvement is typical with Lambert-Eaton Myasthenic's Syndrome. Ann Neurol 2003;53:270.

Evoli A, Minisci C, Di Schino C, et al. Thymoma in patients with MG: characteristics and long-term outcome. Neurology 2002;59:1844.

Scherer K, Bedlack RS, Simel DL. Does this patient have myasthenia gravis? JAMA 2005;293:1906.

Vincent A, Bowen J, Newsom-Davis J, et al. Seronegative generalised myasthenia gravis: clinical features, antibodies, and their targets. Lancet Nuerol 2003;2:99.

Diminished Visual Acuity and Eye Pain

ID/CC: 22-year-old right-handed woman presents with diminished visual acuity and eye pain.

HPI: Over the last 3 days, BS has noticed that she has had difficulty seeing in her left eye. She went to an optometrist for an increased prescription in that eye. She has also had new headaches over her left face. She describes eye pain, that is worse on movement. She has not had any fevers, nausea, or vomiting. She has not had any diplopia or loss of vision.

PMHx: None

PSHx: Tonsillectomy

Meds: Oral contraceptive pills

All: NKDA

SHx: Lifelong nonsmoker, college student, single, lives in an apartment with two roommates

FHx: HTN and migraine headaches in her mother.

Neuro Hx: None

THOUGHT QUESTIONS

- What are neurologic causes of eye pain?
- What are ophthalmologic causes of eye pain?
- What signs will you look for on examination to aid in diagnosis?
- What is the differential diagnosis for optic neuritis?

Eye pain and vision loss can be a difficult problem to sort out because the "lesion" can be ophthalmologic, neurologic, or both. It is important for any patient to have a complete eye history and examination. Patients should be asked about trauma, lacrimation, foreign body sensation, seasonal allergies and photophobia. A complete exam includes full visual acuity testing, funduscopic examination, and slit-lamp examination. Intraocular pressures should be measured. The patient should be evaluated for allergic eye disease, iritis, uveitis, retinal detachment, corneal abrasions, and glaucoma to name just a few important diagnoses.

Neurologic examination should include a full mental status examination, cranial nerve, strength, sensation, reflex, and coordination testing in addition to the eye examination. With regard to the neuro-ophthalmologic examination, special attention should be given to visual field testing, extraocular movements, visual acuity, color perception, and pupillary testing.

Optic neuritis is inflammation of the optic nerve, and patients will present often present with diminished acuity, eye pain that is worse on movement and diminished color vision. On examination, patients may reveal the Marcus Gunn pupil. This abnormality is caused by an afferent pupillary defect. When light is shown to the affected eye, the pupil response may be minimal to none. However, it will react consensually and constrict when light is shown to the unaffected eye. This is because there is bilateral efferent control of the pupillary response. Because of the inflammation, the affected eye is not receiving the stimulus. However, when the unaffected eye is given the stimulus, both eyes will constrict. Funduscopic examination may demonstrate disc pallor as well.

Optic neuritis is most commonly associated with multiple sclerosis; however, a number of other inflammatory processes can cause inflammation of the nerve. They include Lyme's disease, tuberculosis, syphilis, HIV, hepatitis, herpes simplex, cytomegalovirus, and sarcoid.

CASE CONTINUED

VS: Temp 98.6°F BP 110/70 HR 76 RR 16

PE: Normal, well appearing woman.

Neuro: MSE: alert and oriented times 4, MMSE 30/30. CN II–XII: intact. Normal extraocular eye movements and full visual fields.

Visual acuity was 20/40 in the right eye and 20/100 in the left eye. Afferent pupillary defect was present in the left eye. There was significant disc pallor in the left eye on funduscopic examination. There was no nystagmus. Motor and coordination: normal bulk and strength throughout.

Reflexes: 2+ throughout. No Babinski signs present.

Sensory: Intact to light touch, pinprick, vibration and temperature throughout

Gait: Normal posture, stride, speed, and pivot turns. No ataxia, intact tandem gait

 QUESTIONS

56-1. Which cells in the CNS make myelin?
   A. Schwann cells
   B. Oligodendrocytes
   C. Astrocytes
   D. Microglia
   E. Ependymal cells

56-2. Which race is most predisposed to optic neuritis?
   A. African American
   B. East Asian
   C. Hispanic
   D. South Asian
   E. Caucasian

56-3. From which of the following cranial nuclei do the efferent fibers of the pupillary reflex originate?
   A. Abducens nucleus
   B. Oculomotor nucleus
   C. Edinger-Westphal
   D. Facial nucleus
   E. Main sensory nucleus of V

56-4. Which of the following CSF tests are often positive in patients with multiple sclerosis?
   A. Oligoclonal bands
   B. Angiotensin-converting enzyme
   C. IgA levels
   D. Prolactin
   E. Acid-fast stain

ANSWERS

56-1. B. Oligodendrocytes make the myelin that coats axons in the CNS. Schwann cells play a similar role in the PNS. Astrocytes are neuronal cells that are "supporting" cells and help to modulate electrolytes and neurotransmission in the synaptic space. Microglia are involved in the immune response in the CNS, and ependymal cells serve as part of the lining around the CSF.

56-2. E. Caucasians, especially those of northern European descent, are several times more likely to develop optic neuritis than individuals of African or Asian descent. In general, there is an increasing prevalence of demyelinating disease as the distance from the equator increases.

56-3. C. The efferent arc of the pupillary reflex originates from the Edinger-Westphal nucleus. Parasympathetic fibers from this nucleus mediate pupillary constriction in response to a light stimulus. The abducens nucleus is in the pons and controls abduction of the eye. The oculomotor nucleus has several subnuclei; however, it also controls many extraocular movements and has eyelid innervation as well. The facial nucleus controls the muscles of facial strength. The main sensory nucleus of CNV is responsible for facial sensation.

56-4. A. Patients with a high degree of clinical certainty for multiple sclerosis often have oligoclonal bands in the CSF. However, there can be both false positives and false negatives. Angiotensin-converting enzyme (ACE) levels are for sarcoid, prolactin levels are drawn rarely to distinguish seizure from pseudoseizure, and acid-fast stains are done to aid with the diagnosis of tuberculosis.

ADDITIONAL SUGGESTED READING

Beck RW, Smith CH, Gal RL, et al. Neurologic impairment 10 years after optic neuritis. Arch Neurol 2004;61:1386.

Beck RW, Trobe JD, Moke PS, et al. High- and low-risk profiles for the development of multiple sclerosis within 10 years after optic neuritis: experience of the optic neuritis treatment trial. Arch Ophthalmol 2003;121:944.

Pirko I, Blauwet LK, Lesnick TG, et al. The natural history of recurrent optic neuritis. Arch Neurol 2004;61:1401.

Left-Sided Facial Droop

ID/CC: A 45-year-old man with facial asymmetry.

HPI: BP is a 45-year-old man who presented to his primary care physician, complaining of facial asymmetry. Three days ago he developed pain behind his left ear. On the day prior to presentation, his smile looked crooked. He then noticed difficulty eating, with food dribbling out of the left corner of the mouth and inability to close his left eye. Because of progressive symptoms and no improvement, he drove in to see his doctor, worried that he might have had a stroke.

PMHx: Negative

PSHx: Negative

Meds: None

All: NKDA

SHx: Married, engineer employed in the high-tech industry

PE: Gen: Normal

VS: Normal

On neurologic examination, mental status was normal. Speech was mildly dysarthric. Cranial nerve examination notable for the following: the left nasolabial fold was less prominent. When asked to smile, the left corner of the mouth did not move as well as the right. He could not close his left eye. The left eyeball appeared to roll upwards when the eyes were closed. The left side of his forehead did not wrinkle as well as the right with upward gaze. The left platysma was weaker than the right. Hearing and taste were normal.

The remainder of his neurologic examination was normal.

THOUGHT QUESTIONS

▪ What type of a lesion does the patient have?
▪ How will you proceed with your evaluation?

The key to determining the type of lesion that the patient has, and then arriving at a differential diagnosis, is to localize where the lesion is. Is this an UMN lesion or a lower motor lesion causing facial weakness?

The origin of fibers controlling motor function of the face is in the primary motor cortex in the precentral gyrus. Fibers originating here course via the internal capsule, cerebral peduncle in the midbrain. Most fibers cross to the contralateral side in the pons and there end in the facial nucleus. The dorsal portion of the facial nerve nucleus controls the upper third of the face, while the ventral portion controls the lower two thirds of the face.

Motor control of the upper portion of the face has bilateral supranuclear input. Therefore with an UMN lesion, facial muscles in the upper third of the face are spared because of intact innervation from the unaffected hemisphere. Examination will show weakness involving the lower portion of the face, (e.g., eye closure will be spared), and with voluntary smiling, the affected side will droop.

In a LMN lesion, all motor fibers going to the ipsilateral muscles are affected, resulting in weakness involving the entire half of the face.

This patient therefore has a LMN lesion.

The usual work-up for a patient presenting with an LMN type of facial weakness consists of a careful history and neurologic examination. If the facial weakness is deemed to be of an LMN pattern and there is no obvious cause, the patient may be observed clinically and a battery of tests is not required at the outset. The natural course of this process, in a large proportion of cases, is gradual recovery (partial or full) over the next few weeks.

Failure to show improvement should prompt a work-up to determine etiology. Nature of work-up will depend upon factors in the history that would predispose the patient to a facial palsy. For instance, a history of travel to Lyme-endemic areas would require that a Lyme titer be obtained, and possibly a gadolinium enhanced MRI scan of the brain and CSF study (Fig. 57-1).

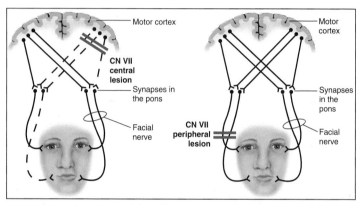

FIGURE 57-1   CN VII—Peripheral Lesion. Peripheral nerve damage to CN VII paralyzes the entire right side of the face, including the forehead. (*From Bickley LS, Szilagyi P. Bates' Guide to PE and History Taking, 8th Ed. Philadelphia: Lippincott, Williams & Wilkins, 2003.*)

CASE CONTINUED

Labs: CBC, electrolytes, blood glucose: WNL

A diagnosis of Bell's palsy was made. The patient was discharged from the ED and asked to follow up with his primary care physician. Over the next 3 weeks, he made a gradual recovery.

QUESTIONS

57-1. What is the significance of hearing/taste abnormality with LMN facial weakness?
- A. Associated with more severe weakness
- B. Helps in localizing lesion along course of the nerve
- C. Both
- D. Neither

57-2. What conditions are associated with LMN facial palsy?
A. Diabetes
B. Pregnancy
C. Herpes zoster infection
D. Lyme disease
E. All of the above

57-3. The following drugs are used in the treatment of Bell's palsy:
A. Phenytoin
B. Prednisone
C. Propranolol
D. Pyridoxine
E. Phenobarbital

57-4. What is Bell phenomenon?
A. Eyeballs rolling upwards with eye closure
B. Inability to close the eye ipsilateral to the weak side
C. Idiopathic facial weakness
D. None of the above

 ANSWERS

57-1. B. The facial nerve gives off branches during its course, and specific symptoms may have value in localizing a lesion along the course of the facial nerve. Lesions outside the stylomastoid foramen present with weakness as described in this case. Lesions in the facial canal proximal to the chorda tympani will result in alteration of taste to the anterior two thirds of the tongue. A lesion more proximal in the facial canal will produce, in addition, hyperacusis because of involvement of the nerve to the stapedius muscle. A lesion proximal to the geniculate ganglion may result in decreased tearing. Lesions at the cerebellopontine angle cause some degree of dysfunction in the vestibulocochlear nerve (eighth cranial nerve).

57-2. E. Table 57-1 outlines etiologies of LMN pattern. The most common etiology is an idiopathic facial palsy, commonly referred to as Bell's palsy, after Graham Bell who described the entity in the late 1800s.

TABLE 57-1 Causes of Lower Motor Neuron Facial Palsy

Idiopathic
Diabetes mellitus
Pregnancy
Trauma
Skull fractures
Birth trauma (forceps) in neonates
Tumor (especially cerebellopontine angle tumors)
Infections
Lyme disease
Herpes infections
Infections involving structures along the facial nerve course
Ramsay-Hunt syndrome
Granulomatous disease
Sarcoid
Congenital
Toxic
Lead poisoning
Guillain-Barré syndrome
Acute intermittent porphyria

57-3. B. The role of steroids in the treatment of Bell palsy is unclear. Some advocate that steroids may hasten recovery when used early in the course of the illness. When used, prednisone is given at a dose of 40 to 60 mg/day and tapered over 10 to 14 days. A course of acyclovir may also be used, if herpes is suspected as the causative agent.

57-4. A. Bell phenomenon is a physiologic response of the eyes to eye closure. With eyelid closure the eyeballs roll upwards because of relaxation of the inferior recti and contraction of the superior recti. In a patient with Bell palsy, this is easily seen as the eyelids do not approximate with eye closure on the weak side.

ADDITIONAL SUGGESTED READING

Benatar M, Edlow J. The spectrum of cranial neuropathy in patients with Bell's palsy. Arch Intern Med 2004;164:2383.

Kress BP, Griesbeck F, Efinger K, et al. Bell's palsy: what is the prognostic value of measurements of signal intensity increases with contrast enhancement on MRI? Neuroradiology 2002;44:428.

Sweeney CJ, Gilden DH. Ramsay Hunt syndrome. J Neurol Neurosurg Psychiatry 2001;71:149.

X

Patients Who Present with an Abnormal Head

Microcephaly

 ID/CC: 8-month-old infant with a small head circumference

HPI: MC is an 8-month-old infant who is evaluated for small head size. The small head circumference was noticed at birth, but was thought to be proportionate to his birth weight. Despite steady weight gain postnatally, there was no concomitant head growth. In addition he is developmentally delayed. He has not begun rolling over, and is not able to sit at the time of his evaluation. His eye contact is poor, and he does not turn his head to sounds. He coos and makes gurgling sounds, but not necessarily in response to parents' or other familiar voices. He has not begun saying any monosyllabic words yet.

PMHx: Cardiac murmur at birth, thought to be secondary to a patent ductus arteriosus (PDA), resolved spontaneously

Meds: Multivitamin drops

All: None

FHx: Noncontributory

SHx: First child. History of one first-trimester miscarriage in mother 6 months prior to conceiving this baby. Maternal age 19 years.

PE: Weight 6.8 kg, length: 60 cm. Head circumference 39.5 cm. General examination: unremarkable.

Neuro: Mental status: Awake, irritable, and generally dull appearance. Makes poor eye contact. Cranial nerves: Pupils equally reactive. Does not fix and follow objects with eyes. Funduscopic examination shows pale optic discs and areas of pigmentation on the retina.

Face: Symmetric. No acoustic blink.

Motor: Increased muscle tone in all limbs, particularly legs and trunk. Moves all limbs.

Reflexes: Brisk bilaterally, with few beats of clonus at ankles

Plantars: Extensor bilaterally

THOUGHT QUESTIONS

- Where is the lesion (UMN or LMN)?
- What other information will be useful in the differential diagnosis?

The history and examination suggest global developmental delay (i.e., in all areas of development). The infant's examination is notable for increased muscle tone (spasticity) and hyperreflexia. The poor visual tracking suggests poor visual acuity, possibly even blindness. Similarly, the lack of an acoustic blink reflex (reflex blinking to loud sound) is suggestive of poor hearing. All these findings in the context of microcephaly (head circumference <2 standard deviations from the mean) point to a disorder of cerebral origin. It is likely to be a diffuse process, given the variety of modalities affected.

Also, that the microcephaly was present at birth, and that the infant was small at birth (intrauterine growth retardation) suggest that the pathologic process began prenatally. Further information that will be useful in the differential diagnosis and in determining the etiology of the child's microcephaly and global delay is that pertaining to risk factors for this child for developmental delay (see questions below). Commonly assessed information includes: details regarding maternal health during pregnancy, gestation at which delivery occurred, complications in the neonatal period, and family history of neurologic disease.

CASE CONTINUED

The child was born at 38 weeks gestation. Birth weight was 1.9 kg and head circumference was 31.5 cm. Pregnancy was notable for poor prenatal care. The infant's mother presented in labor at 38 weeks. The infant spent 2 weeks in the intensive care nursery, for "feeding and growing" issues, but left the hospital prior to a complete work-up. He was then lost to follow-up until presentation.

Work-up: A CT scan of the brain was obtained (Fig. 58-1).

A hearing assessment shows bilateral sensorineural hearing loss.

An ophthalmologic examination shows bilateral optic atrophy and a retinal picture consistent with chorioretinitis.

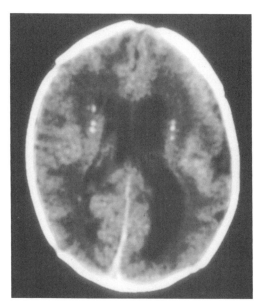

FIGURE **58-1**
CT scan (axial image) shows periventricular calcifications and atrophy. (*Image courtesy of Dr. JS Hahn, Stanford University Medical Center, Stanford, California.*)

THOUGHT QUESTION

■ How does the work-up help with the diagnosis further?

      The CT shows calcifications that strongly suggest an intrauterine infection as the etiology for the infant's condition. The sensorineural hearing loss and retinopathy further confirm the diagnosis. The pattern of calcifications is suggestive of intrauterine CMV infection. This can be confirmed by a urine culture to isolate the virus.

QUESTIONS

58-1. The term toxoplasmosis, other agents, rubella, cyto-megalovirus, herpes simplex (TORCH) infection includes which pathogen:
- A. Toxocara
- B. Rubella
- C. *Candida albicans*
- D. Adenovirus

58-2. Which of the following conditions is more often associated with macrocephaly than microcephaly?
- A. Intrauterine TORCH infections
- B. Cerebral dysgenesis
- C. Perinatal strokes
- D. Storage disorders

58-3. Urine culture in congenital CMV infection stays positive for what duration after birth?
- A. 3 months
- B. 6 months
- C. 9 months
- D. 12 months

58-4. Eye abnormalities in intra uterine infections include:
- A. Cataracts
- B. Retinitis
- C. Both
- D. Neither

ANSWERS

58-1. B. The term TORCH is an acronym for toxoplasma, other (syphilis, listeria, adenovirus, varicella, enterovirus), rubella, cytomegalovirus, herpes simplex. These are organisms that cause congenital infections in a fetus, and several specific clinical syndromes are identified because of these organisms.

58-2. D. Microcephaly can be present in any condition that adversely affects brain growth and development. Intra uterine infections, perinatal hypoxic/ischemic insults, and cerebral malformations are all commonly associated with macrocephaly. In storage disorders (mucopolysaccharidosis, Niemann-Pick's disease,

Tay Sachs' disease, etc.) it is common to see a larger-than-normal head circumference, usually related to intracranial accumulation of abnormal metabolic products.

The differential diagnosis of microcephaly includes:

- Hypoxic-ischemic encephalopathy
- Cerebral dysgenesis
- Inborn errors of metabolism
- Maternal phenylketonuria
- HIV
- Intra uterine infections (TORCH)

58-3. D. CMV particles are shed in the urine of affected infants for as long as 12 months (even longer periods of excretion have been reported), making it convenient to test babies for congenital CMV. Recovery of the virus within the first 3 weeks of life is considered diagnostic of congenital infection. At later times isolation of the virus cannot differentiate between congenital and postnatal infection, and therefore must be used in conjunction with serologic tests.

58-4. C. Both cataracts and chorioretinitis can be seen in intrauterine infections such as rubella, CMV, and toxoplasmosis.

 ADDITIONAL SUGGESTED READING

Fowler KB, Stagno S, Pass RF. Maternal immunity and prevention of congenital cytomegalovirus infection. JAMA 2003;289:1008.

Guerra B, Lazzarotto T, Quarta S, et al. Prenatal diagnosis of symptomatic congenital cytomegalovirus infection. Am J Obstet Gynecol 2000;183:476.

Hamprecht K, Maschmann J, Vochem M, et al. Epidemiology of transmission of cytomegalovirus from mother to preterm infant by breastfeeding. Lancet 2001;357:513.

CASE **59**

Macrocephaly

CC/ID: 6-month-old male infant with a larger than normal head

HPI: HY is a 6-month-old male infant, evaluated for a large head circumference. At his 6-month well-child visit, his head circumference was "off the charts." He was born following an unremarkable pregnancy. Labor was induced at 41 weeks, and delivery was uneventful. At birth he weighed 7 lbs 14 oz (3.6 kg) and was discharged home with his mother. Other than mild jaundice in the first week, his neonatal period was unremarkable. Developmental history reveals that he began holding his head well without support by 4$^1/_2$ months of age. He rolls over in both directions, and sits with support. He reaches for toys, and coos. HY's parents think his vision is okay, but cannot provide a more detailed history.

PMHx: Mild gastroesophageal reflux in early infancy, improving

Meds: None

All: None

FHx: Unremarkable

SHx: 3-year-old sibling, father is an engineer, mother is a homemaker.

THOUGHT QUESTION

- What is the differential diagnosis of a "large head"?

"A large head" or macrocephaly refers to head circumference greater than two standard deviations above the mean.

Differential diagnosis includes the following:

- hydrocephalus
- structural malformations (megalencephaly, posterior fossa)
- intracranial space-occupying lesions
- neurocutaneous disorders
- metabolic diseases
- thickening of skull
- familial macrocephaly

Hydrocephalus: increase in CSF, with dilatation of the ventricles

Structural brain malformations involving the posterior fossa, e.g., Dandy-Walker malformation

Megalencephaly: enlargement of cerebral hemispheres with underlying structural abnormality (dysgenesis)

Intracranial space occupying lesions such as tumors, chronic subdural hematoma, vascular malformations. A high index of suspicion should be maintained for intracranial space occupying lesions if macrocephaly is of short duration/acquired, rapidly progressing, and accompanied by other neurologic deficits.

Metabolic's diseases such as Canavan or Alexander's disease, storage disorders such as Tay-Sachs' disease, or the mucopolysaccharidoses

Neurocutaneous' diseases such as neurofibromatosis.

Thickening of the skull as is seen in diseases like achondroplasia.

Familial macrocephaly, where a child has a large head circumference, and either one of his parents has a large head too. Usually autosomal dominant. No developmental or neurologic abnormalities (except minimal clumsiness) are present on history or exam.

 CASE CONTINUED

PE: Weight 7.5 kg, head circumference: 48 cm (>95th percentile). Father's head circumference: 57 cm (50th to 75th percentile) cm, mother's head circumference: 55.5 cm (50th to 75th percentile). Previous head circumference: Birth, 35 cm; 2 months, 39.5 cm; 4 months, 44 cm.

HEENT: Anterior fontanel wide open, posterior fontanel open, coronal suture spilt. No cranial bruit.

CV: No murmur, lungs: clear, no organomegaly

Neuro: Alert, made eye contact with examiner. Pupils equally reactive. Tracked objects horizontally with ease, but upgaze was limited. At rest, it looked like he was looking down frequently. Face symmetric. No difficulty with sucking or swallowing.

Motor: Mild hypertonia in lower extremities. Reflexes brisk at knees and ankles. Upper extremity reflexes normal.

Work-up: MRI scan of the brain (Fig. 59-1).

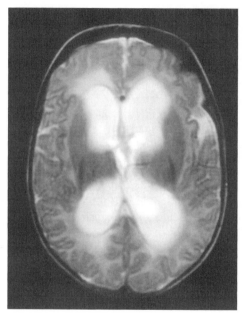

FIGURE **59-1**
MRI scan (axial T2 image) shows dilated ventricles. (*Image provided by Stanford University Medical Center, Stanford, California.*)

THOUGHT QUESTION

- How do his examination and MRI scan further help with the diagnosis?

Key findings on his examination are macrocephaly that cannot be explained as familial, widening of cranial sutures, limitation of upgaze (descriptively termed "sun-setting"), and mild spasticity and hyperreflexia in his lower extremities. The child is not hypotonic, which argues against a leukoencephalopathy such as Alexander's or

Canavan's disease. The MRI scan also does not show abnormal white matter, which would be present in these metabolic diseases. What is more likely is a structural abnormality involving the posterior fossa or hydrocephalus. The CT scan shows dilatation of the lateral ventricles, third ventricle, and normal posterior fossa structures. This picture is consistent with hydrocephalus.

QUESTIONS

59-1. By what age should the anterior and posterior fontanels close, respectively?
- A. 4 months and 4 months
- B. 18 months and 2 months
- C. 2 months and birth
- D. 3 months and 9 months

59-2. Hydrocephalus may be seen with:
- A. Cerebral malformations
- B. Following meningitis
- C. Neural tube defects
- D. None of the above
- E. All of the above

59-3. The foramen of Monro connects:
- A. Lateral ventricles
- B. Lateral ventricles and third ventricle
- C. Third ventricle and fourth ventricle
- D. Fourth ventricle and subarachnoid space

59-4. Definitive treatment of hydrocephalus involves:
- A. LP
- B. Treatment with diuretics
- C. Ventriculoperitoneal shunt
- D. Steroids

ANSWERS

59-1. B. The anterior fontanel ("soft spot") is usually open at birth, and closes between 9 and 18 months of age. The posterior fontanel closes by 6 to 8 weeks after birth.

59-2. E. Hydrocephalus is seen with a variety of conditions. Communicating hydrocephalus is because of impaired absorption of CSF or excessive CSF production and may be seen following meningitis or with tumors of the choroids plexus. Noncommunicating hydrocephalus is because of obstruction of flow of CSF from the ventricles to the subarachnoid space, and is seen in neural tube defects, various cerebral malformations (e.g., holoprosencephaly), and stenosis of the aqueduct of Sylvius.

59-3. A. The lateral ventricles connect in the midline to the third ventricle via the foramen of Monro. The third ventricle is connected to the fourth ventricle via the aqueduct of Sylvius. The fourth ventricle opens into the subarachnoid space via the foramen of Magendie in the midline and the foramen of Luschka laterally ("M" midline, "L" lateral).

59-4. C. Treatment of hydrocephalus involves providing an alternate route for CSF drainage. This is achieved by placing a shunt that drains CSF from the ventricles into another body cavity. Various types of ventricular shunts are used. Ventriculoperitoneal shunting is the most commonly employed method. Diuretics and steroids are not particularly useful in treating hydrocephalus.

 ADDITIONAL SUGGESTED READING

Custer DA, Vezina LG, Vaught DR, et al. Neurodevelopmental and neuroimaging correlates in nonsyndromal microcephalic children. J Dev Behav Pediatr 2000;21:12.

Misshapen Head

ID/CC: 8-month-old male infant who presents with a misshapen head.

HPI: DP is 8 months old. He was born via a normal spontaneous vaginal delivery (NSVD) without complications and went home on the second day of life. Approximately 2 months ago, the patient's mother began to notice that his head appeared oddly shaped. She is concerned that his misshapen head is related to the delivery. The patient was evaluated by the pediatrician and subsequently referred to neurosurgery.

PMHx: None

PSHx: None

Immunizations: Up to date

Meds: None

All: NKDA

FHx: No significant family history

PE/Neuro: The anterior fontanel is soft. The OFC is 50th percentile. The left forehead is bulging. The left ear is slightly anterior and inferior to the right ear. There is no palpable ridge across either the sagittal, coronal, or lambdoid sutures.

THOUGHT QUESTIONS

- What is the patient's differential diagnosis?
- Is this mother's concern regarding the delivery leading to this problem justifiable?
- What is meant by the term craniosynostosis?
- What is the difference between craniosynostosis and deformational plagiocephaly?

The differential diagnosis includes craniosynostosis versus deformational plagiocephaly (e.g., lazy lambdoid).

The mother's concerns regarding birth trauma are not justifiable. Although birth trauma may result in misshapen head, it is usually transient. The sutures of the skull remain open and as the child's head grows, the shape changes appropriately.

The term craniosynostosis refers to the premature closure of the sutures of the cranium resulting in abnormal shape of the skull as it grows. There are several types of craniosynostosis. The most common type involves the sagittal suture and is known as dolichocephaly or scaphocephaly. Synostosis of the coronal suture may be unilateral (plagiocephaly) or bilateral (brachycephaly). Craniosynostosis of the coronal suture is associated with both Crouzon's syndrome and Apert's syndrome. Trigonocephaly refers to synostosis of the metopic suture. Premature closure of all sutures is known as pansynostosis.

Unlike craniosynostosis, deformational plagiocephaly refers to the misshapen head that is secondary to positional flattening versus premature closure of the cranial sutures.

CASE CONTINUED

The radiograph demonstrates normal lucency across all sutures. The CT confirms the patency of the sutures.

THOUGHT QUESTIONS

- What is your diagnosis at this time?
- What course of action would you consider?

        As the radiographs demonstrate open sutures, craniosynostosis is omitted from the diagnosis. The PE and history support a diagnosis of deformational plagiocephaly. As noted above, the misshapen head results from prolonged placement of the infant's head in a particular position that causes flattening. Over time the result is the noted misshapen head with shearing of the ears.

Had the sutures been prematurely closed, surgical intervention might have been indicated. As the diagnosis is deformational plagiocephaly, such intervention is deferred. Other treatment options are discussed in detail below.

 ## CASE CONTINUED

The patient is fitted with a helmet and the infant is prevented from lying on the affected side. Within weeks, there is improvement.

 ## QUESTIONS

60-1. Which of the following types of craniosynostosis is usually genetic?
- A. Brachycephaly
- B. Plagiocephaly
- C. Scaphocephaly
- D. Dolichocephaly

60-2. Trigonocephaly refers to the premature closure of which of the following sutures?
- A. Sagittal
- B. Coronal
- C. Metopic
- D. Lambdoid

60-3. Deformational plagiocephaly is associated with which of the following?
- A. Cardiac abnormalities
- B. Syndactyly
- C. Mental retardation
- D. None of the above

60-4. What is the initial treatment for deformational plagiocephaly?
- A. Surgical intervention
- B. Anticonvulsant therapy
- C. Changing the sleeping position of the child
- D. None of the above

ANSWERS

60-1. A. Brachycephaly, premature closure of bilateral coronal sutures, is usually genetic and is associated with both Apert and Crouzon's syndrome. Both of these syndromes are autosomal dominant (AD). Crouzon's syndrome is the most common craniofacial syndrome associated with midface hypoplasia, mental retardation, and an increased incidence of hydrocephalus. Apert's syndrome is the second most common craniofacial syndrome. It is associated with syndactyly; mental retardation; deafness; gastrointestinal (GI), genitourinary (GU), and cardiac abnormalities; frontal encephalocele; and vertebral and skeletal abnormalities. Plagiocephaly refers to unilateral premature closure of coronal suture (coronal synostosis). Scaphocephaly and dolichocephaly refer to premature closure of the sagittal suture (sagittal synostosis).

60-2. C. Trigonocephaly refers to premature closure of the metopic suture and results in a pointed forehead with a ridge located in the midline. Sagittal synostosis results in a boat shaped head with frontal bossing. Coronal synostosis may be unilateral or bilateral. When unilateral, the forehead is flattened on the affected side and appears flat, and the supraorbital margin is higher on the affected side. When bilateral, the forehead is broad and flattened. This is usually associated with Crouzon's or Apert's syndrome.

60-3. D. All of the above choices are associated with Apert's syndrome, not deformational plagiocephaly. Apert's syndrome is also associated with deafness, GI and GU abnormalities, frontal encephalocele, and vertebral and skeletal abnormalities. Deformational plagiocephaly results from positional flattening.

60-4. C. Deformational plagiocephaly is initially treated with conservative measures. The family is advised to change the sleeping position of the head. In some cases, the infant is helmeted for a period of weeks to months. There is no indication for the use of anticonvulsant therapy.

 ADDITIONAL SUGGESTED READING

Lajeunie E, Catala M, Renier D. Craniosynostosis: from a clinical description to an understanding of bone formation of the skull. Childs Nerv Syst 1999;15:676.

XI

REVIEW Q&A

Questions

Directions: Each of the numbered items or incomplete statements in this section is followed by answers or by completions of the statement. Select the *one* lettered answer or completion that is best in each case.

1. A 30-year-old man with no significant past medical history presents with confusion, lethargy, fever, and stiff neck. The lumbar puncture reveals a CSF analysis that is remarkable for 200 RBC, 100 WBC, most of which are lymphocytes, and protein of 150 mg/dL. An MRI reveals hyperintensity along the medial temporal lobe. Which of the following medications would be most appropriate for this patient?
  A. Dexamethasone
  B. Vancomycin
  C. Ceftriaxone
  D. Acyclovir
  E. Ampicillin

2. A 40-year-old woman presented to her primary care physician with 2 months of headache, fatigue, and malaise. She has been sexually active and denies using any barrier protection. She had no deficits on examination. An LP was performed, and her opening pressure was 300 mm. She had 20 WBC, which were mostly mononuclear cells, 0 RBC, and normal glucose and protein. Which of the following tests on the CSF is most likely to reveal the diagnosis?
  A. Angiotensin-converting enzyme (ACE) level
  B. Lactate
  C. India ink
  D. Herpes simplex virus PCR
  E. Venereal Disease Research Laboratory (VDRL)

3. A 20-year-old college student presents with one day of headache, stiff neck, and photophobia. On examination, he is febrile, has nuchal rigidity, and is found to have a petechial rash on his trunk and lower extremities. Overnight, he becomes hypotensive and dies from septic shock the following morning. Which of the following agents should be used for chemoprophylaxis for his classmates living in the adjacent dormitories?

A. Rifampin
B. Bactrim
C. Prednisone
D. Acyclovir
E. Penicillin

4. Several weeks after a root canal, a 65-year-old woman presents with a left frontal headache. She complained of being increasingly tired over the previous 3 days. On examination, she was afebrile and had a right pronator drift and right leg weakness. A head CT with contrast showed a ring-enhancing lesion with surrounding edema. What is the next step in management?

A. Antibiotics alone
B. Antibiotics and surgery
C. Lumbar puncture
D. Steroids
E. Mannitol

5. A 40-year-old man has had progressive difficulty with his memory over the course of several months. He has become has less interactive, had difficulty with his concentration, and occasionally seemed very anxious. On examination, he has no focal cranial nerve findings or weakness. When the examiner claps his hands loudly, the patient exhibits a dramatic startle response. He has no chorea or athetosis. An MRI of his head shows increased signal bilaterally in his caudate and putamen. What is the most likely diagnosis?

A. Herpes encephalitis
B. Cryptococcal meningitis
C. Huntington's disease
D. ALS
E. Jakob-Creutzfeldt's disease

6. A 70-year-old man with a history of hypertension, hyperlipidemia, and CAD develops new onset headache followed by right face, arm, and leg weakness. He is brought to the emergency room, where his initial labs show an INR of 1.1 and platelets of 275,000. His blood pressure is 200/100. A head CT and CT angiogram are performed and reveal hemorrhage. Which of the following is the most likely location and cause of his bleed?

A. Left frontal lobe, amyloid angiopathy
B. Left frontal lobe, coagulopathy
C. Left putamen, AVM
D. Left putamen, hypertension
E. Left midbrain, aneurysm

7. A 27-year-old woman presents with gait difficulty after visiting a chiropractor. She has an MRI/MRA that shows a vertebral artery dissection. She is diagnosed with a Wallenberg stroke. Which of the following examination findings would you expect to see in this patient?

    A. Arm weakness
    B. Leg weakness
    C. Horner's syndrome
    D. Light touch deficits
    E. Visual field cut

8. A 40-year-old patient has developed new migraines over the course of the previous 5 years. In the last 2 months, he has noticed significant difficulty with his hearing and has had confirmed bilateral auditory dysfunction. Today, he presents with right face and arm weakness and is found to have a stroke in his left parietal lobe. On history, he reports stroke younger than the age of 50 years in three other family members, two of which also had hearing loss. This patient likely has a genetic abnormality affecting which of the following?

    A. Mitochondria
    B. Vascular smooth muscle
    C. Coagulation cascade
    D. Microtubules
    E. Golgi apparatus

9. A 35-year-old man presents to the ED after a tonic-clonic seizure. He has had a mild posterior headache for 2 days. However, he has no other symptoms and on examination, he is lethargic but has no focal neurologic deficits. He has had no fevers and a CT head of his head is negative. A MRI and MR venogram are ordered, which reveal a filling defect in the venous study in the superior sagittal sinus. The MRI shows 2 cm of parasagittal blood in the right posterior parietal lobe. What is the most appropriate step in management?

    A. Surgery
    B. Observation
    C. Avoidance of any antiplatelet agents
    D. Heparin
    E. Aspirin

10. A 70-year-old woman has had 2 weeks of sore throat, facial pain, and runny nose. Her primary care physician (PCP) diagnoses her with sinusitis. Over the last 2 days, she has had increasing headache, and she presents to the ED. On examination, she is found to have proptosis of her right eye, right sided ptosis and miosis, asymmetric facial sensation in the ophthalmic portion of the trigeminal nerve, and an abduction deficit of her right eye. Where can these deficits be localized?

A. Superior cervical ganglion of internal carotid artery
B. Cavernous sinus
C. Pons
D. Medulla
E. Midbrain

11. A 32-year-old woman on oral contraceptives presents with a global aphasia and right face and arm weakness. She is found to have a left middle cerebral artery stroke. Her left lower extremity is also swollen, and ultrasound studies reveal a deep vein thrombosis (DVT). If the blood clot in her leg was the source of the stroke, what cardiac abnormality would cause an arterial embolus?

A. Tricuspid valve atresia
B. Tricuspid valve stenosis
C. Right atrial myxoma
D. Pulmonary valve stenosis
E. Patent foramen ovale

12. A 60-year-old man with a history of hypertension presents to the ED with headache and mild confusion. His blood was 210/120, his toxicology screen was positive for cocaine, and he was diagnosed with hypertensive encephalopathy. He was given IV metoprolol tartrate (Lopressor) to lower his blood pressure; but instead, it increased to 240/130. What was the mechanism of action to explain this effect?

A. Unopposed α receptor mediated vasoconstriction
B. Activation of the β_1 receptors
C. Central α antagonist
D. Vasopressin-like effects
E. Cross-activation of dopamine receptors

13. A 78-year-old man with mitral stenosis and hypertension presents with a left homonomous hemianopia. The MRI shows a right posterior cerebral artery distribution stroke. As part of his stroke work-up, Holter recording shows that he has intermittent atrial fibrillation and is placed on warfarin sodium (Coumadin). What is the mechanism of action of this medication?

A. Inhibition of Vitamin A recycling
B. Inhibition of Vitamin D recycling
C. Inhibition of Vitamin K recycling
D. Inhibition of Vitamin E recycling
E. Inhibition of Vitamin B6 recycling

14. A 27-year-old attorney presents to the ED with an abnormal sensation over the legs for the past 3 days. The sensation seems to be moving up her legs. Initially, she has no other symptoms or signs except for some mild back pain. After 2 days, her voice has become more nasal, and she has a foot drop. On examination, she has absent reflexes in her lower extremities. On further questioning, she reports that she had an episode of abdominal discomfort 2 weeks ago. What is the underlying pathophysiology for the most likely disease process?

- A. Antibodies to acetylcholine receptors
- B. Immune-based demyelination of axons
- C. Primary motor neuron dysfunction
- D. Mutation in kinesin and dynein transport systems
- E. Glycogen storage

15. A 50-year-old woman with 2 months of weight loss and mild headache presents with shaking of her right arm for the last month. The episodes last for 5 to 10 minutes and occur several times a day. They have been more frequent recently. She has no other symptoms during the episode, and there is no change in her level of consciousness. What type of seizure is this patient having?

- A. Simple partial seizure
- B. Complex partial seizure
- C. Tonic-clonic seizure
- D. Myoclonic seizure
- E. Absence seizure

16. A 35-year-old woman with no medical history presents to the ED with the worst headache of her life. Over the next few hours, she falls into a coma and a CT scan of her head reveals a large hemorrhage. The CT angiogram shows multiple aneurysms. Her condition worsens, and despite aggressive measures, she passes away. The autopsy reveals multiple cysts in her kidney which have been found in several of her family members as well. What is the inheritance pattern for the disorder that likely caused both her cysts and aneurysms?

- A. Autosomal dominant
- B. Autosomal recessive
- C. X-linked dominant
- D. X-linked recessive
- E. Co-dominant

17. A 53-year-old man with word-finding difficulty presents to clinic. He is complaining of an episode where he had shaking of his right upper and lower extremity that lasted for five minutes. An

EEG shows several spikes in the left hemisphere. A CT of his head shows a mass lesion that is suspicious for glioblastoma multiforme. His episode of shaking was most likely a seizure. Which of the following is an important precaution for the patient to take?

    A. Avoid caffeine
    B. Avoid high altitudes
    C. Avoid roller coasters
    D. Avoid airplane travel
    E. Avoid driving

18. A 30-year-old man with a history of alcohol abuse presents to the ED after a tonic clonic seizure. His last drink was 48 to 72 hours ago, and it is thought that his seizure is from alcohol withdrawal. His head CT is negative for any acute pathology. What is the best medication for this patient to prevent further seizures?

    A. Dilantin
    B. Phenobarbital
    C. Valproic acid
    D. No long term medication; alcohol cessation
    E. Limit consumption to 3 to 4 drinks per day

19. A 71-year-old woman with dementia is brought to the ED because of a sudden change in mental status. She appears to be weak on her right arm and leg, and a head CT reveals a large lobar hemorrhage in her left frontal lobe that is suspicious for amyloid angiopathy. It is decided that there is no indication for surgical intervention, so she will be medically managed. She is loaded with phenytoin sodium (Dilantin) in the ED for seizure prophylaxis. What is the mechanism of action of Dilantin?

    A. Calcium channel blocker
    B. Magnesium channel blocker
    C. Sodium channel blocker
    D. Potassium channel blocker
    E. Glutamate antagonist

20. A 60-year-old man with hypertension presents with a left homonomous hemianopia and is found to have a right posterior cerebral artery stroke. His inpatient work-up reveals atrial fibrillation by Holter monitor, and he is started on warfarin sodium (Coumadin) for secondary stroke prevention. What is the mechanism of action for this medication?

    A. Inhibition of Vitamin A recycling
    B. Inhibition of Vitamin K recycling
    C. Inhibition of Vitamin D recycling
    D. Inhibition of Vitamin E recycling
    E. Inhibition of Vitamin B6 recycling

21. A 70-year-old woman with a recent upper respiratory inf[...] and sinusitis presents with headache, right eye proptosis, dip[...] on right lateral gaze, diminished right facial sensation to pin[...] and right eye ptosis and miosis. Where is the most likely lesion[...]

A. Pons
B. Midbrain
C. Medulla
D. Cavernous sinus
E. Hypothalamus

22. A 40-year-old woman presents to the neurology clinic wi[...] numbness and tingling in her left hand and right foot. She is als[...] mildly weak in the same distribution, and you feel that she may hav[...] a polyneuropathy or mononeuritis multiplex. You send off severa[...] laboratory studies. On further questioning, you discover that she ha[...] a rash on her arm 2 years ago with central clearing followed by[...] arthralgias for several months. Which of the organisms is most likely[...] responsible for the patient's presentation?

A. *Haemophilus influenzae*
B. *Campylobaceter jejuni*
C. CMV
D. *Listeria monocytogenes*
E. *Borrelia burgdorferi*

23. A 15-year-old patient presents to neurology clinic with several months of difficulty with his gait that has been getting progressively worse. On examination, he has profound dysmetria of all four extremities and significant loss of vibration and position sense. He also has an upgoing toe and occasional incontinence. He was recently diagnosed with diabetes, and after several months of dyspnea on exertion, ECG revealed an ejection fraction of 40%. Which of the following genes is responsible for his presentation?

A. Frataxin
B. Huntington
C. Parkin
D. ApoE
E. Neurofibromin

24. A 44-year-old woman presents with progressive difficulty combing her hair and climbing steps for several months. On examination, she is found to have symmetric 3/5 weakness in her proximal muscles in both her upper and lower extremities. Her skin examination reveals nodules over her elbows and knuckles as well as a dark rash over her eyelids. Her creatinine kinase levels are

has a negative Tensilon test. What is the most

myopathy
tomyositis
ıyositis

r-old boy presents to neurology clinic because of weak-
unning, and jumping. He is seen to have pseudohyper-
ıis calf muscles and uses his arms to push himself off the
examination, he is found to have proximal greater than
remity weakness. His CK is markedly elevated. There are
other man members of his family that have had similar
ms and early death. What is the genetic defect and inheri-
ıattern of the disease?

. Dystrophin, autosomal dominant
ı. Dystrophin, autosomal recessive
ⁿ. Dystrophin, X-linked recessive
D. Spectrin, autosomal dominant
E. Spectrin, autosomal recessive

. A 75-year-old man presents with 6 months of progressive dys-
ıagia. For the last 2 months, he has become more hoarse and his
bice is more nasal. He has had negative ENT and gastrointestinal
GI) evaluations and has been referred to neurology clinic. Atop
the differential diagnosis is MG and ALS. In order to differentiate
between the competing diagnoses, a Tensilon test is performed
and is positive. Which of the following describes the basis for the
Tensilon test?

A. It stimulates acetylcholine release from the presynaptic
   neuron.
B. It acts as an agonist on the post-synaptic acetylcholine
   receptor.
C. It prevents degradation within the presynaptic neuron.
D. It inhibits the acetylcholinesterase inhibitor.
E. It recruits and acts on non-acetylcholine receptors on the
   postsynaptic neuron.

27. An 8-year-old boy presents to clinic after having several
months of fatigue and cold intolerance. He is found to have a TSH
of 10, and he is diagnosed with hypothyroidism. An MRI shows a
mass in the suprasellar region that is likely to be a craniopharyn-
gioma. Visual field examination reveals a bitemporal hemianopia.

Where along the visual pathway is the most likely location for compression by the mass?
- A. Both optic nerves
- B. Thalamus
- C. Midbrain
- D. Hypothalamus
- E. Optic chiasm

28. A 70-year-old man with a 100-pack per year of smoking history presents with 2 months of weakness, shortness of breath, and bilateral ptosis. He has a chest CT and is found to have a circumscribed mass. Which of the following sites is the location of the lesion causing his ptosis and weakness?
- A. Postsynaptic acetylcholine receptor
- B. Presynaptic calcium channels
- C. Synaptic acetylcholinesterase
- D. LMN
- E. Muscle

29. A 28-year-old man presents to clinic with diminished urine output and an abdominal ultrasound shows a large renal mass that is found to be clear cell carcinoma, by biopsy. Six months later, he is found to have diminished acuity and pain in his right eye. Further work-up reveals a retinal hemangioma. What syndrome should this patient be evaluated for?
- A. Von Recklinghausen's disease
- B. Pompe's disease
- C. Von Hippel-Lindau's disease
- D. Gaucher's disease
- E. Leber hereditary optic neuropathy

30. A 16-year-old African-American boy presents to the ED with 3 hours of left-sided weakness. On examination, he is not able to demonstrate how to turn a key into a door or how he would salute a soldier; has a left homonomous hemianopia; and left face, arm, and leg weakness. He is found to have a right MCA stroke by MRI. Which of the following should be most included as part of the stroke work-up in this young patient?
- A. Notch mutation
- B. Anti-nuclear antibody
- C. Renal magnetic resonance angiogram
- D. Skin biopsy
- E. Hemoglobin electrophoresis

31. A 12-year-old boy is admitted to the ICU in respiratory failure after several months of muscle weakness. He was found to have an enlarged liver, and an ECG showed an ejection fraction of 35%. Metabolic testing revealed a deficiency in acid maltase. Which of the following disorders does this child have?

A. Pompe's disease
B. Tay-Sachs' disease
C. Danon's disease
D. Von Gierke's disease
E. Hers' disease
F. Anderson's disease
G. Gaucher'd disease
H. Fanconi's syndrome
I. McArdle's disease
J. Niemann-Pick's disease

32. A 20-year-old college student who used to run and play tennis in high school presents to clinic because of several months of fatigue, myalgias, and exercise intolerance. He reports that he feels like his muscles are swelling occasionally. He reports that he has had trouble running the same distance he used to without becoming very fatigued; however, if he stops to rest for several minutes, he is able to go another distance at full strength before becoming tired again. This patient should be evaluated for which of the following?

A. Pompe's disease
B. Tay-Sachs' disease
C. Danon's disease
D. Von Gierke's disease
E. Hers' disease
F. Anderson's disease
G. Gaucher's disease
H. Fancon's disease
I. McArdle's disease
J. Niemann-Pick's disease

33. A 50-year-old woman with a history of asthma diagnosed 2 years ago presents to the neurology clinic with facial weakness. She reports not being able to smile for the last 2 to 3 weeks. On examination, she is not able to wrinkle her forehead, close her eyes tight, puff out her cheeks, or smile broadly on either side of her face. A review of her records shows a chest radiograph done 1 year ago that showed hilar lymphadenopathy. Which of the following diagnoses does this patient have?

A. Lyme's disease
B. Guillain Barré
C. Sarcoid
D. Tuberculosis

E. Syphilis
F. Lupus
G. Wegner
H. Multiple sclerosis
I. Mobius' syndrome
J. Bilateral pontine strokes

34. A 72-year-old woman with a history of glioblastoma multiforme presents to the emergency department after a witnessed generalized tonic-clonic seizure. In the ED, she has a fever to 101.5, a blood pressure of 90/60 mm Hg, and a heart rate of 110. She receives normal saline 1L IV bolus, ceftriaxone 1g IV, phenytoin sodium (Dilantin) 1g IV, and vancomycin 1g IV. She has another seizure and receives lorazepam 2 mg IV. Her heart rate drops precipitously to 52 and her blood pressure dips to 80/55 mm Hg. What is the most likely cause of the change in her hemodynamics?
A. Sepsis
B. Seizure
C. Dilantin
D. Lorazepam
E. Ceftriaxone
F. Vancomycin

35. A 28-year-old man IV drug user presents with fever, left calf pain, and weight loss over the past 3 weeks. On examination, the patient has an irregular cardiac rhythm, a loud murmur, petechiae under his fingernails, and left calf pain. Blood cultures are drawn and an ultrasound is obtained that reveals a left leg deep venous thrombosis. Before starting anticoagulation for the deep vein thrombosis (DVT), what study should be obtained?
A. Transesophageal ECG
B. Chest CT with contrast
C. Brain MRI
D. Brain angiogram
E. Electrocardiogram

36. A 45-year-old woman presents with a left thalamic stroke. During the work-up of her stroke, it is found that she has elevated anticardiolipin immunoglobulin (IgG) antibodies. Which of the following data would *not* prompt you to start the patient on long-term anticoagulation?
A. Ultrasound showing DVT
B. Evidence of atrial fibrillation
C. Evidence of amyloid angiopathy on MRI
D. Positive repeat anticardiolipin IgG antibodies 2 months later

37. A 14-year-old boy with a history of congenital heart disease status post-transplant is brought to the ED as a result of 3 days of worsening confusion. The patient had been started on phenytoin sodium (Dilantin) 2 weeks prior for a generalized tonic-clonic seizure. He also takes cyclosporine, trimethoprim-sulfamethoxazole (Bactrim), and multivitamin. In the ED, his blood pressure is 180/100 mm Hg, and an MRI reveals T2 hyperintense foci in the bilateral occipital lobes. What is the most likely cause of the patient's presentation?
  A. Dilantin
  B. Cyclosporine
  C. Bactrim
  D. Hypoxia
  E. Acute rejection

38. A 30-year-old obese woman with a history of childhood asthma presents to the neurology clinic as a result of 2 months of refractory headaches without other symptoms. Examination reveals papilledema and a subtle left cranial nerve VI palsy. Which of the following is the most appropriate next step in the work-up and treatment?
  A. Noncontrast CT scan
  B. Referral to neuro-ophthalmology
  C. MRI with venography
  D. Lumbar puncture
  E. Trial of acetazolamide treatment

39. A 44-year-old woman with a history of COPD and hypertension presents to urgent care clinic with headache and low-grade fever. She recently had a diarrheal illness with some fevers, but improved spontaneously. She has been taking ibuprofen for headaches she developed during the gastrointestinal (GI) illness. Her examination is normal. You refer her to the emergency room, where CT scan is unremarkable and lumbar puncture reveals normal glucose, slightly elevated protein, and a lymphocytic pleocytosis (40 WBC, 95% lymphs). What is the most likely cause of her illness?
  A. Enterovirus
  B. Meningococcus
  C. Herpes simplex virus 1
  D. Epstein-Barr virus
  E. Ibuprofen

40. A 75-year-old man presents to neurology clinic with recurrent burning pain in the area of his left chest, axilla, and back. He notes that the problem started soon after he developed a red rash over that area 2 months prior. The pain has become such that he avoids cold environments where he must wear heavy clothes, as the clothes exacerbate the pain. He denies any headaches, joint aches, or tick bites. What is the most appropriate treatment?

- A. Gabapentin
- B. Acyclovir
- C. Ceftriaxone
- D. Doxycycline
- E. Prednisone

41. A 29-year-old physician presents to your office because for the past three weeks he has had pain and weakness in his left fourth and fifth digits. These symptoms have limited his ability to play the piano, which he usually does on a daily basis. What is the most likely site of the problem?

- A. Medial cord of the brachial plexus
- B. Radial nerve at the elbow
- C. Ulnar nerve at the elbow
- D. Median nerve at the elbow
- E. Median nerve at the wrist

42. A 35-year-old woman presents to the ED after waking up with left arm and leg weakness. On examination, she has 3/5 strength in her left arm and leg, as well as a slight left facial droop. On further history, she has a long history of severe migraines, sometimes involving neurologic symptoms such as weakness or numbness, which usually resolve completely. Her mother died from a stroke in her 40s, and she has several siblings with migraines and early strokes. She has five children, the oldest of which is 18 and also has migraines. MRI obtained in the ED reveals an acute stroke in the right internal capsule, as well as multiple periventricular and sub-cortical T2 hyperintensities, especially in the bilateral temporal poles. The defect involved in this pathology is most likely:

- A. Notch-3 gene mutation leading to small vessel occlusion
- B. Oligoclonal autoantibodies leading to demyelination in the CNS
- C. Mitochondrial cytochrome C-1 activity leading to failure of energy metabolism
- D. Antibodies to phospholipid leading to hypercoagulability

43. A 65-year-old man with a history of hypertension, borderline diabetes, and alcohol abuse presents with numbness and tingling in his feet that has progressed over the past few months. On examination, he has impairments in vibration and position sense in his lower extremities to his knees, and in his fingertips bilaterally.

Which of the following would *not* be a useful part of the immediate work-up of this patient?
- A. TSH
- B. Serum protein electrophoresis
- C. EMG and nerve conduction studies
- D. Hemoglobin A1C
- E. Vitamin B12 level
- F. Urinalysis
- G. MRI spine
- H. ESR
- I. ANA

44. A 67-year-old woman presents to the emergency room after being found unresponsive and quadriplegic. On careful examination, you find that the patient has intact vertical gaze and can make eye movements in response to command, but all other movement is absent. What is the most likely location of the lesion?
- A. Medullary pyramids
- B. Bilateral MCA
- C. High cervical cord
- D. Ventral pons
- E. Midbrain

45. An 18-month-old boy is brought to the office for fever and rhinorrhea. On examination, his temperature is 102.7 and his examination is otherwise unremarkable. As you are finishing the exam, the patient has a 30-second generalized tonic-clonic seizure followed by sleepiness. After a few minutes, you re-examine him. He is easily aroused, has no nuchal rigidity or neurologic findings. His mother tells you that she thinks his father had a seizure when he was an infant, but there is no history of seizures in the family beyond childhood. What is the most appropriate course of action?
- A. Obtain brain MRI
- B. Perform lumbar puncture
- C. Check urinalysis, blood chemistries, and CBC
- D. Obtain sleep-deprived EEG
- E. Prescribe prophylactic Phenobarbital
- F. Recommend supportive measures for URI

46. A 65-year-old woman Russian immigrant presents to the ED with 3 weeks of low-grade fever, intermittent nausea and vomiting, and headache, with 1 day of confusion. Further history from her daughter reveals that the patient has had pulmonary tuberculosis in the past treated in Russia. Examination is remarkable for temperature of 100.3°F, delirium, and a left cranial nerve VI palsy. MRI shows

enhancement of the basal meninges with mild hydrocephalus. Lumbar puncture would be expected to show which of the following:
A. Mildly elevated opening pressure
B. Elevated protein at 250 mg/dL
C. Low glucose at 35 mg/dL
D. Mixed neutrophilic and lymphocytic pleocytosis (300 WBC, 35% polys, 55% lymphs, 10% monos)
E. Positive acid fast bacilli smear
F. All of the above

47. A 33-year-old man with HIV presents to clinic with 3 months of worsening cognitive function and depressed mood. Serologic testing, lumbar puncture, and brain imaging rule out opportunistic CNS infections, and he is given a diagnosis of HIV-associated dementia. Which of the following is *not* characteristic of this syndrome?
A. Psychomotor slowing
B. Memory impairments
C. Movement disorders
D. Seizures
E. Improves with antiretroviral therapy

48. A 74-year-old man with a history of hypertension, CAD, and COPD presents to the ED after developing slurred speech and weakness of his left hand manifested as dropping his spoon repeatedly. On exam, he has intact language, slurred speech, left facial droop, and left hand weakness, with full strength in the left upper arm and left leg and no sensory deficits. What is the most likely etiology of his deficit?
A. Cardioembolic event
B. Large-vessel embolic event
C. Large-vessel occlusion
D. Small-vessel occlusion
E. Vasospasm
F. None of the above

49. An 84-year-old woman with a history of hypertension and diabetes presents with right sided-weakness and speech difficulties. Which of the following would *not* help localize the lesion to the cortex?
A. Dysarthria
B. Aphasia
C. Apraxia
D. Neglect
E. Homonymous hemianopsia
F. Agnosia

50. A 3-year-old boy presents to the ED after waking up from a nap and being unable to stand. Further history reveals recent chicken pox infection. On exam, the patient is unable to sit up unassisted because of swaying (truncal ataxia). Neurologic examination is otherwise normal, including normal reflexes. What is the most likely cause of the symptoms?

- A. Varicella meningitis
- B. Hydrocephalus
- C. Cerebellar tumor
- D. Postinfectious cerebellitis
- E. Miller-Fisher's syndrome
- F. Ataxia telangiectasia
- G. Chiari malformation type-2
- H. Friedreich ataxia

51. A 30-year-old woman with no significant medical history presents to the clinic with 3 months of intermittent headache and left face pain. The pain is a shooting sensation on the left side of her face that comes and goes, but is often followed by a headache. She has tried aspirin, acetaminophen, and ibuprofen without benefit. Cranial nerve examination is normal. Which of the following is unlikely to be a cause of her symptoms?

- A. Giant cell arteritis
- B. Multiple sclerosis
- C. Cerebellopontine angle schwannoma
- D. Brainstem meningioma
- E. Microvascular compression

52. A 65-year-old man with a history of CAD presents to the office with several months of fluctuating cognitive function, with several recent falls. Over the past few weeks, his wife reports that he has been having some visual hallucinations. On examination, the patient has mildly impaired short-term memory and some constriction of affect, normal cranial nerves, some mild rigidity and bradykinesia, but no tremor. CT scan is remarkable only for some mild atrophy. Which of the following is the most likely diagnosis?

- A. Alzheimer's disease
- B. Lewy-body dementia
- C. Pick's disease
- D. Corticobasal ganglionic degeneration
- E. Normal pressure hydrocephalus
- F. Progressive supranuclear palsy
- G. Vitamin B12 deficiency
- H. Neurosyphilis
- I. Wilson's disease

53. An 84-year-old woman comes to the emergency after a fall. No traumatic injury is found, but on exam the patient is not oriented to time or place. On further history, her daughter reports 6 months of worsening cognitive function. She had attributed it to old age and has not had a work-up. Which of the following studies would *not* be indicated at this time?

A. TSH
B. Vitamin B12 level
C. RPR
D. Brain MRI
E. Lumbar puncture

54. A 50-year-old right-handed woman presents with complaint of headache and left hand weakness. On further history, she reports that her left hand sometimes "does its own thing" independently of what she is doing with her right hand. She finds that she has trouble setting the table using both hands because her left hand does not coordinate with her right. Where would you expect to find a lesion on neuro-imaging?

A. Right parietal cortex
B. Left frontal cortex
C. Right thalamus
D. Right frontal cortex
E. Corpus callosum

55. A 45-year-old woman with a history of migraines presents to the ED with the acute onset of left face, arm, and leg weakness. On further history, the weakness seemed to spread from her face down to her arm and leg over a period of 30 minutes. She then developed a bifrontal headache. On exam, she has a left facial droop and 4/5 strength in her left arm and leg. MRI shows no diffusion abnormality and MR angiography shows no stenosis of any cerebral vessels. What class of medication is contraindicated in this patient?

A. β-blockers
B. Triptans
C. Calcium channel blockers
D. NSAIDs
E. Tricyclic acid antidepressants

56. A 5-year-old boy presents to the clinic with headache, vomiting, and unsteady gait. On examination, the patient has papilledema, truncal ataxia, and increased reflexes. MRI reveals an enhancing mass in the vermis of the cerebellum. Which of the following statements is *not* characteristic of this tumor?

A. It is typically slow-growing.
B. It is a primitive neuroectodermal tumor.
C. It is the most common primary brain tumor with onset during infancy.
D. It often causes hydrocephalus by obstructing the fourth ventricle.
E. It is treated with surgery, radiation, and chemotherapy.

57. A 65-year-old man with a history of COPD and CAD presents with COPD exacerbation and receives IV steroids. He subsequently develops pneumonia and sepsis requiring intubation and vasopressors. He has a long course in the ICU, but as his infection improves he is found to be weak in all his extremities. He is able to follow some commands, but cannot lift his arms or legs off the bed. His reflexes are diminished. Which of the following would likely be most helpful in narrowing the differential?

A. Serum acetylcholine receptor antibody titre
B. MRI cervical spine with and without contrast
C. MRI brain
D. Lumbar puncture
E. EMG/nerve conduction studies

58. A 55-year-old woman with a history of epilepsy is admitted with status epilepticus. She initially receives lorazepam followed by phenytoin IV, but the phenytoin is discontinued because of hypotension and bradycardia. She then receives valproic acid IV, which is continued along with phenytoin per NG tube. She also receives vancomycin IV and levofloxacin per NGT. Three days later, laboratory studies reveal hyperammonemia without abnormalities in her liver enzymes or bilirubin. What is the most likely cause?

A. Lorazepam
B. Phenytoin
C. Valproic acid
D. Vancomycin
E. Levofloxacin

59. A 35-year-old woman undergoes surgery under general anesthesia. Her surgery is uncomplicated, but in the PACU she develops fever to 104°F and rigidity. Laboratory studies reveal a metabolic acidosis and myoglobinuria. Which of the following is *not* part of treatment for this condition?

A. Dantrolene infusion
B. Induced hypothermia
C. Bicarbonate infusion
D. IV fluid administration
E. Furosemide infusion
F. Atropine infusion

60. A 67-year-old woman comes to your office for evaluation of symptoms she first noticed 2 to 3 months prior. She describes a distressing, uncomfortable feeling in her legs as if she "needs to shake them." It is worse when she goes to bed at night. It is not painful, but causes her much distress and frustration as she has trouble falling asleep because of the sensation deep in her legs. Once she moves her legs, the sensation goes away. She is having the symptoms every night. Her husband has noticed that she has also had increased jerking of her muscles during sleep. What is the most appropriate treatment in this case?
A. Pramipexole
B. Oxycodone
C. Clonazepam
D. Zolpidem
E. Diphenhydramine
F. Quetiapine

61. A 19-year-old man presents with trouble swallowing and speaking. On eye examination, he has bilateral brown corneal rings. His spleen is enlarged. On neurologic examination, he has dysarthria, dysphagia, rigidity, and ataxia. Laboratory tests show abnormal liver function tests. Which of the following is not characteristic of this disease?
A. It always affects the liver prior to the brain.
B. In the brain, it affects primarily the caudate, putamen, cortex, and cerebellum.
C. It can cause dementia and psychosis.
D. It is inherited in autosomal recessive pattern.
E. It is reversible.

62. A 56-year-old man with a history of hypertension presents with left arm and leg tingling for the prior 3 days. On examination, he has no subjective sensory loss but reports paresthesias throughout his left arm and leg. Cervical MRI reveals an enhancing lesion in the cervical cord. Brain MRI reveals multiple nonenhancing T2 lesions in the periventricular white matter. Based on the radiographic findings, you suspect multiple sclerosis (MS). Because of his older age and man gender,

you perform a lumbar to help assess the possibility of MS. Which of the following would be inconsistent with a diagnosis of MS?
A. Oligoclonal bands
B. Elevated IgG index
C. Lymphocytic pleocytosis with 75 cells/µL
D. Normal opening pressure
E. Mildly elevated albumin
F. Normal glucose

63. A 25-year-old woman with chronic headaches and normal head imaging presents to clinic for elective lumbar puncture to assess for idiopathic intracranial hypertension. What is the most common adverse event from a lumbar puncture?
A. Infection
B. Epidural hematoma
C. Temporary nerve damage
D. Headache
E. Transtentorial herniation

64. A 23-year-old man presents with headache and fever for 2 days followed by rapid decline in mental status. In the ED, he is started immediately on ceftriaxone, vancomycin, ampicillin, and acyclovir. The patient is intubated. Head CT reveals global edema with uncal herniation. The patient is hyperventilated and given mannitol infusion without change in mental status. He is taken to the operating room for emergent craniectomy. Following surgery, off all sedation, the patient remains unresponsive. Which of the following is *not* required to declare brain death?
A. Known irreversible cause
B. Exclusion of metabolic abnormalities such as severe acidosis or electrolyte disturbances
C. Normothermia
D. Negative toxicology screen
E. Observation period for changes
F. Absent cranial nerve reflexes
G. Absent spontaneous breathing as proven by apnea test
H. Absent cerebral response to noxious stimuli
I. EEG showing absence of electrocerebral activity

65. A previously healthy 55-year-old woman presents with acute onset of unsteadiness leading to a fall. In the ED, trauma is ruled out but the patient is unable to stand without falling. Examination reveals nystagmus and truncal ataxia. MRI is normal. Lumbar puncture reveals normal protein, glucose, and cell counts. CSF cultures and PCR are negative, but anti-Yo antibodies are positive. Which of the following studies would likely not be helpful?

- A. Mammogram
- B. CT scan with contrast of chest, abdomen, and pelvis
- C. Pelvic ultrasound
- D. Cerebellar biopsy
- E. PET scan

66. A 40-year-old man from Greece presents with right hand resting tremor, difficulty initiating movements, and frequent falls. On examination, he has marked cogwheel rigidity in his right wrist, but also in his right leg. Further history reveals that his father and three of his siblings have had similar symptoms. Which of the following genes or gene products is associated with this disease?

- A. α synuclein
- B. Notch-3
- C. SOD1
- D. Huntingtin
- E. DYT1

67. A 35-year-old adopted man has just been given the diagnosis of Huntington's disease. He asks you the probability that he has passed the disease on to his 5-year-old son. In order to answer him, you must know that Huntington's disease has which of the following inheritance patterns?

- A. Autosomal dominant
- B. Autosomal recessive
- C. X-linked dominant
- D. X-linked recessive
- E. Mitochondrial inheritance

68. A 15-year-old boy presents with progressive generalized dystonia, depression, and jaundice. Ophthalmologic examination reveals brown deposits in the outer rim of the cornea. Which of the following laboratory abnormalities would most likely be found?

- A. Low serum aminotransferase
- B. Low serum ceruloplasmin
- C. Low serum nonceruloplasmin bound copper
- D. Low urine copper excretion
- E. Low hepatic copper concentration

69. A 35-year-old woman presents to the ED with the worst headache of her life, with sudden onset 2 hours earlier. CT reveals subarachnoid hemorrhage and CTA shows a berry aneurysm. She is taken to the operating room for surgical clipping and then transferred to the neurologic ICU. Prophylaxis by which of the following medications can help to diminish the incidence and severity of vasospasm, a frequent complication of aneurysmal SAH?

   A. Acetazoleamide
   B. Propanolol
   C. Captopril
   D. Hydrochlorothiazide
   E. Nimodipine

70. An 80-year-old woman presents with a headache over her right temple. On further questioning, she reports new onset of blurry vision. Which of the following laboratory tests is likely to be the most revealing?

   A. WBC count
   B. Lipase
   C. ANA
   D. ESR
   E. TSH

71. If the patient in the case above presented with a seizure in addition to her previously mentioned complaints, which of the following diagnoses would become much more likely.

   A. Stroke
   B. Uncal herniation
   C. Venous sinus thrombosis
   D. Migraine
   E. Multiple sclerosis

72. A 24-year-old woman presents with café-au-lait spots, axillary freckling, and iris hamartomas. History reveals that her mother had similar findings, as well as a brain tumor of unknown character. Which CNS tumor is commonly seen in this autosomal dominant syndrome?

   A. Astrocytoma
   B. Optic glioma
   C. Lymphoma
   D. Acoustic neuroma
   E. Pineal tumor

73. A 75-year-old man is referred by his PCP for behavioral changes including a new ritual for daily hygiene and inappropriate sexual comments, as well as word-finding problems. According to his family, the symptoms have been worsening over the past 3 years. Which of the following types of dementia is characterized by gradual and progressive behavioral change and language dysfunction?

A. Alzheimer's disease
B. Huntington's disease
C. Normal pressure hydrocephalus
D. Vascular dementia
E. Fronto-temporal dementia

74. A 68-year-old woman with idiopathic Parkinson's disease for 15 years is seen in follow-up because of concerns among her family regarding her memory and decision making. On examination, she has significant impairments in executive functioning, set shifting, and episodic memory. Which of the following pathologic correlates would most likely be seen in this case?
A. Senile plaques
B. Lewy bodies
C. Amyloid deposition
D. Trinucleotide expansion
E. Neurofibrillary tangles

75. A 45-year-old HIV-positive woman on three-drug antiretroviral therapy with a CD4 count of 250 cells/μL and a viral load of less than 50,000 copies/mL is seen in follow-up. Her boyfriend notes that she has withdrawn from her prior social activities. Otherwise, her mood is good, she has no sleep disturbance, and she has a good appetite. On examination, she has trouble reciting the months of the year backwards and doing mathematical word problems. Which of the following medications would be indicated at this time?
A. Methylphenidate
B. Zoloft
C. Imipramine
D. Valproic acid
E. Lithium

76. An 8-month-old baby girl is brought to your office by her parents, who are concerned that she is not yet standing on her own. She is able to assume a sitting position on her own, take a few steps holding onto her parents with both hands, and stand with assistance but not on her own. What age is the normal milestone for a child to be able to stand alone?
A. 3 to 6 months
B. 6 to 9 months
C. 9 to 12 months
D. 12 to 15 months
E. 5 to 18 months

77. A 62-year-old man with a history of hypertension, diabetes, hypercholesterolemia, and smoking presents for a routine physical.

On further history, you learn that his father suffered a stroke at age 55 years. On examination, he has no carotid bruits, normal heart sounds, and no neurologic findings. Laboratory screening reveals an elevated homocysteine level. ECG shows normal sinus rhythm. Which of the following modifiable risk factors is most important for primary prevention of ischemic stroke?

   A. Hypertension
   B. Smoking cessation
   C. Diabetes
   D. Hyperhomocysteinemia
   E. Hyperlipidemia

78. A 62-year-old woman is brought to the ED by her daughter, who found the patient confused and acting strange. In the ED, she is alert with normal vitals. Neurologic examination reveals she is disoriented and not reliably following commands but has no focal findings. Laboratory studies are sent for basic chemistries, hematology, toxicology, and urinalysis. Which of the following electrolyte abnormalities can be responsible for a change in mental status and confusion?

   A. Low magnesium
   B. High magnesium
   C. High chloride
   D. Low chloride
   E. High calcium

79. A 22-year-old man college student presents to the ED with headache, fever, rash, and drowsiness, worsening over the past 4 hours. The patient is immediately given IV antibiotics and a head CT is obtained which is unremarkable. An LP is performed and shows an opening pressure of 18 cm H_2O, protein of 120, glucose of 15, 4 RBCs, and 100 WBCs (90% PMNs with some bands). In addition to antibiotic administration, which of the following additional therapies has been shown to improve overall neurological outcome in patients with bacterial meningitis?

   A. Intravenous hydration
   B. Steroids
   C. Mannitol
   D. Acetazolamide
   E. Aspirin

80. A 55-year-old man is brought to the ED by his family, who report that he was difficult to arouse from bed this morning. In the ED, he has a blood pressure of 160/90 mm Hg, a heart rate of 100, and an oxygen saturation of 96% on 2-L nasal cannula. You are asked to examine the patient prior to his intubation. As part of your

coma exam, you perform oculocephalic testing. An intact oculo-cephalic response is seen when the patient's eyes:
  A. Move in a conjugate direction away from the direction of head turn
  B. Move in a conjugate direction toward the direction of head turn
  C. Move in the direction of the head turn for only the ipsilateral eye
  D. Move in the direction of the head turn for only the contralateral eye
  E. Move opposite the direction of the head turn for only the ipsilateral eye

81. An 81-year-old man is referred to your clinic for several weeks of unilateral right temporal headache. On history, he reports that he first noticed the pain when combing his hair on the right side. He has noticed over the past few days that his jaw hurts at the end of a meal and he has had episodes of blurry vision. On examination, he has a temperature of 101.2°F and tenderness to palpation over the right temple. Laboratory studies reveal an ESR of 67. What is another laboratory test that can be used in addition to ESR to evaluate for temporal arteritis?
  A. Ferritin
  B. Platelets
  C. Fibrin split products
  D. C-reactive protein
  E. ANA

Answers and Explanations

1. D	**21.** D	**41.** C	**61.** A
2. C	**22.** E	**42.** A	**62.** C
3. A	**23.** A	**43.** G	**63.** D
4. B	**24.** C	**44.** D	**64.** I
5. E	**25.** C	**45.** F	**65.** D
6. D	**26.** D	**46.** F	**66.** A
7. C	**27.** E	**47.** D	**67.** A
8. A	**28.** B	**48.** D	**68.** B
9. D	**29.** C	**49.** D	**69.** E
10. B	**30.** E	**50.** D	**70.** D
11. E	**31.** A	**51.** A	**71.** C
12. A	**32.** I	**52.** B	**72.** B
13. C	**33.** C	**53.** E	**73.** E
14. B	**34.** C	**54.** E	**74.** B
15. A	**35.** D	**55.** B	**75.** A
16. A	**36.** C	**56.** A	**76.** C
17. E	**37.** B	**57.** E	**77.** A
18. D	**38.** C	**58.** C	**78.** E
19. C	**39.** A	**59.** F	**79.** B
20. B	**40.** A	**60.** A	**80.** A
			81. D

1. The answer is **D**. This patient likely has herpes simplex virus encephalitis, given his presentation of acute confusion. The lumbar puncture can reveal many red blood cells and typically has an increased number of lymphocytes and protein. He should be treated with acyclovir, which help to disrupt replication of the virus. Until the Gram stain is negative, and evaluation by HSV polymerase chain reaction is not complete, patients will often need antibiotic therapy to cover bacterial organisms. Ampicillin is used to treat *L. monocytogenes*.

2. The answer is **C**. The most likely diagnosis in this patient is CNS cryptococcus. She has HIV risk factors; however, cryptococcus can present in patients that are not immunocompromised as well. The clinical course is often indolent, without focal neurologic signs. Patients often have an elevated CSF opening pressure greater than 200 mm. India ink staining of the CSF will often show encapsulated yeast forms. Elevated ACE levels are found in sarcoid, but the sensitivity is low. VDRL used to test for neurosyphilis.

3. The answer is **A**. The original patient likely had meningococcal meningitis, which can be a deadly CNS infection. Close contacts, including household members, office workers, and students, have a much higher rate of infection after contact with the affected individual on the order of several hundred-fold compared to the general population. Prophylaxis with rifampin significantly diminishes the rate of attack.

4. The answer is **B**. With the recent history of a dental procedure, a brain abscess has likely complicated the patient's course. The pathogenesis was likely a result of direct extension as opposed to hematogenous spread, commonly seen in patients with endocarditis. Her increasing fatigue is concerning and may be a consequence of significant edema. In the setting of focal findings or signs of increased intracranial pressure, a lumbar puncture is contraindicated. Blood cultures should be drawn and prompt antibiotic therapy initiated. Surgical drainage is indicated for therapy and microbial identification.

5. The answer is **E**. Jakob-Creutzfeldt's is a neurodegenerative disease that are associated with the accumulation of prion proteins. Mental status changes, dementia, and myoclonus are the hallmarks of the disease. Some patients develop some evidence of corticospinal tract injury. A startle response to a loud stimulus is seen in most patients. MRI findings include hyperintensities in the basal ganglia. CSF levels of a protein 14-3-3 can be found in many patients; however, it is not a very sensitive or specific test in all populations. Huntington's disease patients typically have chorea, athetosis, mood and personality changes. ALS is a disease of motor neurons, and patients can present with cranial motor nerve palsies or weakness.

6. The answer is **D**. Hypertensive hemorrhages usually occur in the putamen, thalamus, pons, cerebellum, and cerebral hemispheres. This patient does not have any known coagulopathy, and his platelets are normal. While vascular malformations can cause a bleed in any location, they are much less likely in the above locations in the setting of high blood pressure. Basal ganglia hemorrhages will often cause weakness in the face, arm, and leg since the many fibers of the corticospinal tract have come together in the adjacent internal capsule as they descend. Frontal lobar hemorrhages will often spare the arm or face.

7. The answer is **C**. Patients with Wallenberg's syndrome have an infarction in the lateral medulla. Classically, this is caused by a lesion in the posterior inferior cerebellar artery; however, patient can have a lesion in the vertebral artery as well. Deficits include ptosis, miosis, anhydrosis (Horner's syndrome), ipsilateral facial pain and temperature loss, contralateral body pain and temperature loss, ataxia, dysphagia, and vertigo. Patients typically do not have any motor weakness.

8. The answer is **A**. This patient likely has MELAS, or a syndrome of mitochondrial encephalopathy, lactic acidosis, and stroke. Patients have a defect in the mitochondrial genes encoding tRNA. There a range of other mitochondrial disorders including Leigh's disease, Leber's hereditary optic neuropathy (LHON), myoclonic epilepsy and ragged red fibers (MERRF). Patients can have multiple neurologic symptoms including strokes, seizures, migraines, ataxia, and dementia. High energy organs such as the eye, heart, and gastrointestinal (GI) tract can also be affected.

9. The answer is **D**. For the most part, seizures have a bimodal age of onset. Many structural and congenital causes of seizures present in childhood and adolescence. In the elderly, brain tumors and strokes often serve as an epileptic focus. When patients present in between these peaks, there should be an aggressive search for a new structural lesion, infection, or vascular cause. This patient has venous sinus thrombosis, which can present with headache, focal neurologic deficit, and seizure. Often times, there is secondary ischemia or hemorrhage. However, even in the presence of blood, these patients often need anticoagulation to treat the underlying process.

10. The answer is **B**. This patient has a cavernous sinus thrombosis. It is likely infectious in etiology given her history of antecedent sinus infection. The internal carotid artery and associated sympathetic fibers, cranial nerves III, IV, V1, V2, and VI pass through the sinus.

The sixth cranial nerve is most medial and unprotected in the sinus, and patients often have an abduction deficit of the ipsilateral eye.

11. The answer is **E**. Anywhere from 20% to 30% of the population may have a patent foramen ovale creating a conduit from the right atrium to the left atrium. The presence of this connection can be demonstrated during a cardiac echocardiogram, when agitated saline bubbles are injected intravenously and observed to be crossing into the left atrium. Deep vein thromboses may travel to the heart via the venous circulation and enter the arterial side through a PFO. It is unclear whether closing the PFO results in a lower rate of stroke recurrence.

12. The answer is **A**. Cocaine prevents reuptake of neurotransmitters and increased sympathetic activation of α and β receptors. If a β-blocker is used, then the B_2 receptor mediated vasodilation of peripheral vasculature is blocked, and the α_1 receptor mediated vasoconstriction is "unopposed." The result is an overall increase in blood pressure. For this reason, beta blockers are often avoided for cocaine induced hypertension. Benzodiazepines and direct α antagonists are used instead.

13. The answer is **C**. Factors II, VII, IX, and X are all Vitamin K–dependent factors in the clotting cascade. Activation of this pathway results in the aggregation of fibrin monomers to become fibrin polymers. Coumadin inhibits the process by which Vitamin K is recycled and the process of coagulation is impaired, so the blood is "thinned." One of the main side effects of warfarin sodium (Coumadin) is excess bleeding.

14. The answer is **B**. The patient has Guillain-Barré's syndrome. There are multiple variants of Guillain-Barré, or acute inflammatory demyelinating polyneuropathy. Patients will present with paresthesias, back pain, weakness, cranial nerve deficits, and autonomic symptoms such as blood pressure variability and bladder spasm. A feared complication is respiratory weakness, and patients often need the support of mechanical ventilation. In one to two thirds of patients, an antecedent upper respiratory or gastrointestinal infection is present. *C. jejuni* is the most commonly identified infectious precipitant.

15. The answer is **A**. The patient is a having a simple partial seizure. In some ways, the episodes could be called auras as well because an aura is the part of the seizure that the patient remembers. Otherwise, the seizure is simple because there is no alteration in consciousness. It is partial because there was spread of cortical activity. Simple partial seizures are often caused by structural lesions. A history of weight loss and headaches should raise concerns for a CNS malignancy.

16. The answer is A. There is a known association between autosomal dominant polycystic kidney disease and cerebral aneurysms. Approximately 5% to 10% of patients with ADPKD have cerebral aneurysms; ones that rupture are usually larger and along the MCA.

17. The answer is E. All patients with seizures must be told to avoid driving, typically for 6 months' duration. Because of the unpredictability of seizure control, drivers can be a danger to themselves and others, and patients should receive appropriate counseling. In many states, it is illegal for patients to drive for a certain time period after a seizure.

18. The answer is D. When there is a provocation for the seizure, especially ones that are metabolic- or toxin-related, like alcohol withdrawal or hyponatremia, there is no indication for seizure prophylaxis. All seizure medications have very significant side effects, which should be avoided when possible. The underlying order should be treated, and if there is no evidence of cortical injury or seizure focus, then antiepileptic therapy can be avoided.

19. The answer is C. Phenytoin sodium (Dilantin) has been in clinical use for seizures for over half a century. It works by blocking voltage- dependent sodium channels. This is thought to inhibit depolarization and consequent excitation of neurons.

20. The answer is B. Warfarin sodium (Coumadin) is efficacious for secondary stroke prevention in a limited number of cases. Atrial fibrillation is such an indication. The medication works by inhibiting Vitamin K recycling. Factors II, VII, IX, and X, which are part of the coagulation cascade, use vitamin K as a cofactor. On Coumadin, the cascade does not work as well to create fibrin polymers and clot, and so the blood is "thinned."

21. The answer is D. The patient likely has a cavernous sinus thrombosis. The cavernous sinus contains cranial nerves III, IV, V1, V2, and VI, as well as the internal carotid artery and the sympathetic fibers that accompany the vessel. The sixth nerve is the most medial within the sinus and the most unprotected, so patients will often have diplopia and an ocular abduction deficit. The antecedent history of sinus infection raises the possibility of a septic thrombosis.

22. The answer is E. The patient's neuropathy is most likely a result of Lyme disease. Lyme disease is caused by *B. burgdorferi* through the Ixodes tick vector and has many systemic manifestations.

Neurological manifestation can be divided into early presentations, which include facial palsies, lymphocytic meningitis, and radiculopathy and late disease, which include encephalopathy, transverse myelitis, and peripheral neuropathy. The late disease is usually seropositive.

23. The answer is A. Friedreich's ataxia is an autosomal recessive disorder that usually presents before the age of 25 years and results from a loss of function mutation. It involve a triplet expansion that results in decreased expression of the gene, whose protein product is involved in mitochondrial function. Patients also have cardiomyopathy and diabetes, in addition to neurological disease. Patients may have optic atrophy and pyramidal signs on examination, in addition to ataxia and neuropathy.

24. The answer is C. This patient has a diagnosis of dermatomyositis. Patients usually have proximal greater than distal muscle weakness. Patients may have a scaly lesion over their extensor surfaces; these lesions are known as Gottron nodules. The heliotrope rash is a red eruption that is usually present at the upper eyelids. Muscle enzymes such as CK and aldolase may be elevated, but normal levels do not exclude the diagnosis. The Tensilon test is positive in patients with MG. ALS patients usually have UMN and LMN signs.

25. The answer is C. Dystrophin is part of a glycoprotein complex that stabilizes muscle fibers. Deficiencies in inheritance are transmitted in an X-linked manner. DMD involves a complete deletion of the gene, and Becker muscular dystrophy usually results in a partial deletion. The former presents earlier and is more deadly. Patients often have a co-existing cardiomyopathy and often die of arrhythmias. Gowers sign describes the patient who uses his or her arms to climb up off the floor.

26. The answer is D. Tensilon is edrophonium, a compound that inhibits the acetylcholinesterase present in the synapse. When this enzyme is inhibited, there is more acetylcholine to compete with the antibodies which bind to the acetylcholine receptors. Patients with MG will often temporarily reverse their deficit with this medication.

27. The answer is E. At the point of the optic chiasm the nasal fibers of each optic nerve cross to the contralateral side. The nasal fibers from each eye represent the temporal field of vision of each eye. Lesions in the optic chiasm strike both sets of nasal fibers and disturb the temporal fields of both eyes. Such lesions include craniophargiomas and pituitary adenomas. The optic chiasm sits above the sella turcica, the portion of bone where the pituitary gland lies.

28. The answer is **B**. The patient has LEMS, a paraneoplastic antibody syndrome seen in patients with malignancy, especially lung cancer. The antibody is directed against P-Q type presynaptic voltage gated calcium channels that are involved in synaptic vesicles formation and release. As opposed to MG, there is an incremental response to repetitive nerve stimulation of the compound muscle action potential.

29. The answer is **C**. Von Hippel-Lindau's disease is caused by a gene defect that is transmitted in an autosomal dominant fashion. Patients can have a variety of tumors such as renal cancer, retinal angiomas and pheochromocytomas.

30. The answer is **E**. Patients with sickle cell disease are at a higher risk of stroke because of vaso-occlusive disease and sludging, endothelial injury and development of moyamoya, to name a few. The diagnosis of sickle cell disease is made by peripheral smear and hemoglobin electrophoresis which reveals substitution of valine for glutamic acid in the place of the sixth amino acid of the beta globin chain. Patients with known sickle cell disease can be followed by transcranial Doppler for primary and secondary prevention.

31. The answer is **A**. Pompe's disease is caused by a deficiency in lysosomal acid maltase. Patients present with infantile or juvenile onset forms. The latter is associated with less severe cardiomyopathy. Serum creatine kinase is usually elevated. Diagnosis usually involves muscle biopsy and testing of the enzyme level from the peripheral blood.

32. The answer is **I**. McArdle's disease is a glycogen storage disorder in which there is a deficiency of muscle phosphorylase. It is inherited in an autosomal recessive manner, and patients will often describe a second-wind phenomenon during exercise. CK will often be elevated in these patients. Patients are treated with a high-protein diet and sucrose before any vigorous exercise.

33. The answer is **C**. This patient has a diagnosis of neurosarcoid. Spinal tap would likely reveal elevated lymphocytes and protein. This patient has bilateral facial nerve palsies. Because she has upper and lower facial weakness, she has a LMN weakness, or a "peripheral seventh." The lower part of the face only has unilateral UMN innervation as opposed to the upper part of the face, which has bilateral UMN innervation. Therefore, if the upper and lower face are affected, it must be a LMN lesion. The differential for bilateral seventh nerve palsies is limited and includes tuberculosis, Lyme, and sarcoid. This patient likely has pulmonary sarcoid as well, given her hilar lymphadenopathy.

34. The answer is C. Phenytoin sodium (Dilantin), when given rapidly intravenously, can cause precipitous drops in blood pressure and heart rate. This can usually be avoided by infusing the Dilantin over a longer time period, such as an hour. If any sudden hypotension or bradycardia develops, the infusion should be stopped immediately until the patient is stabilized. Lorazepam can also cause hypotension, but less commonly causes bradycardia. Sepsis, which is a possibility in this case, can also cause hypotension, but the timing of the hemodynamic is more consistent with IV Dilantin administration. Oral Dilantin does not share this potential adverse effect. Seizures more typically cause hypertension, but do not typically cause hemodynamic changes after they have ceased. Ceftriaxone and vancomycin are not known to cause this reaction.

35. The answer is D. The patient's constellation of symptoms and signs is suggestive of bacterial endocarditis. Intravenous drug users are at increased risk. A potential complication of bacterial endocarditis is development of mycotic aneurysms in the CNS vasculature. These are small aneurysms in the arteries of the brain caused by deposits of infectious material in the vascular wall. Such aneurysms are friable and at high risk for rupture, leading to devastating intraparenchymal hemorrhages. They can sometimes be seen on CT or MR angiography, but conventional angiography is the gold standard for diagnosis and can also be used for treatment by targeted embolization of bleeding vessels. If mycotic aneurysm is present on angiography, it might change your decision to anticoagulate this patient in the short term. Medical treatment for mycotic aneurysm is to treat the underlying infection. A transesophageal ECG should be performed to help confirm the diagnosis and extent of cardiac damage, but would not determine the use of anticoagulation.

36. The answer is C. Amyloid angiopathy is associated with lobar intraparenchymal hemorrhages because of friable vessels, and anticoagulation is contraindicated. DVT and atrial fibrillation are both well-established indications for anticoagulation. Antiphospholipid antibody syndrome (APLS) is a syndrome in which antibodies to the phospholipid components of cells lead to a hypercoagulable state. The clinical criteria for the syndrome include evidence of thrombosis and an elevated antiphospholipid antibody titre (anticardiolipin IgM, anticardiolipin IgG, or lupus anticoagulant) at two time points at least 6 weeks apart. A repeat positive IgG in this case would meet the criteria for APLS, the treatment for which is anticoagulation for goal INR 2 to 3.

37. The answer is **B**. The patient likely has the reversible posterior leukoencephalopathy syndrome (RPLS). This is a syndrome of neuro-logic changes associated with neuro-imaging evidence of white matter changes typically in the posterior circulation, which is reversible with correction of the underlying cause. Common presenting symptoms include headache, confusion, visual impairments, and seizures, often associated with acute hypertension. The etiology is thought to be vasogenic edema, to which the posterior circulation is more suscepti-ble. Some identified causes include hypertensive encephalopathy, eclampsia, glomerulonephritis, and use of certain immunosuppressive drugs including cyclosporine and tacrolimus.

38. The answer is **C**. The patient has symptoms and signs of intracranial hypertension. Given that she has had symptoms for the past 2 months and that papilledema takes at least days to weeks to develop, the process has likely been going on for some time. While the most likely diagnosis is idiopathic intracranial hypertension (pseudotumor cerebri), other etiologies should be ruled out, namely mass lesions or cerebral sinus thrombosis. An MRI with venography would reveal whether the ventricles are enlarged, as well as show any mass lesion or sinus thrombosis. If the imaging is unremark-able, a lumbar puncture should be performed to measure the open-ing pressure, which must be elevated (>180 mm H_2O) in order to make the diagnosis of idiopathic intracranial hypertension. Acetazo-lamide, a carbonic anhydrase inhibitor thought to decrease produc-tion of CSF, is sometimes effective in treating this syndrome.

39. The answer is **A**. The findings are suggestive of a viral or aseptic meningitis. The most common cause of aseptic meningitis is enterovirus (echoviruses and coxsackie viruses types A and B). These viruses can also cause diarrhea, among other symptoms. HSV-1 and 2 is another common cause of viral meningitis, which can also cause encephalitis and seizures. The CSF profile can be similar to enterovirus, and HSV PCR should be obtained before attributing the meningitis to other etiologies, as treatment with acyclovir is indicated for HSV. EBV is a less common cause of viral meningitis. NSAIDs such as ibuprofen have been known to rarely cause aseptic meningitis, and these agents should be avoided once aseptic meningitis is identified so that there is no confusion in subsequent evaluations.

40. The answer is **A**. The patient most likely has postherpetic neu-ralgia. Varicella zoster virus can remain latent in dorsal root gan-glia, to be reactivated in states of immune compromise such as old age, HIV, or chemotherapy. Herpes zoster or shingles manifests typ-ically as pain or paresthesias in a dermatomal distribution (most commonly T2–12), followed by painful vesicular rash. In the acute period, acyclovir can shorten the course of the rash and if given within 72 hours of onset, can help prevent postherpetic neuralgia. Steroids in conjunction with acyclovir have also been shown to improve symptoms. This patient is beyond the window of benefit of acyclovir or steroids. Gabapentin has been shown to give some benefit in postherpetic neuralgia.

41. The answer is C. Sensation to the fourth and fifth digits is supplied by the ulnar nerve, which also innervates the wrist flexors, digit 3 and 4 flexors, and most of the interosseous muscles of the hand. Compression of the ulnar nerve at the elbow is the second most common site of nerve compression in the upper extremities (after the carpal tunnel). The ulnar nerve is less commonly affected at the wrist in the ulnar tunnel (Guyon canal).

42. The answer is A. The patient most likely has the CADASIL syndrome (*c*erebral *a*utosomal *d*ominant *a*rteriopathy with *s*ubcortical *i*nfarcts and *l*eukoencephalopathy). Symptoms include migraines, mood disturbances, recurrent strokes, and progressive dementia. MRI typically shows white matter lesions, particularly in the anterior temporal lobes. The defect is a mutation in the *Notch-3* gene, which encodes a transmembrane protein involved with blood vessel development. The defect is inherited in an autosomal dominant pattern.

43. The answer is G. The patient's symptoms and signs are consistent with a metabolic polyneuropathy, rather than a process in the spine. EMG/NCV can help best elucidate whether the process is primarily neuropathic or myopathic, as well as distinguish between polyneuropathy and polyradiculopathy. The most common systemic causes of polyneuropathy are diabetes, critical illness, and late in the course of malignancy.

44. The answer is D. The patient has locked-in syndrome, characterized by quadriplegia and anarthria, with preserved vertical eye movements and consciousness. The syndrome is caused by a lesion in the ventral pons, which disrupts all corticospinal and corticobulbar fibers at the level of cranial nerve IV. The most common etiology is an embolus to the basilar artery, but can also be a result of hemorrhage or trauma.

45. The answer is F. The patient most likely had a simple febrile seizure. Seizures in the setting of fever before the age of 2 years are considered simple febrile seizures if the seizure is not prolonged, there are no signs of developmental or neurological abnormality, no signs of CNS infection, no family history of epilepsy, and a normal exam after the seizure (i.e., not comatose). Family history of febrile seizures is suggestive of this diagnosis, as it is felt to be inherited.

In these cases, no further work-up or treatment is indicated, although patients may have one or two more seizures in the setting of fevers. These are not dangerous and do not typically lead to epilepsy.

46. The answer is F. The patient most likely has tuberculous meningitis. The usual CSF pattern includes normal to elevated opening pressure, elevated protein (sometimes as high as 400 mg/dL), low glucose, and a lymphocytic pleocytosis in the range of 200 to 400 WBC (with PMN predominance earlier in the course). AFB smears are positive in 20% to 30% of cases, but yield increases with repeated LPs. PCR is sometimes helpful if AFB is negative, but is not sensitive enough to rule out TB if negative. If TB is suspected, specific treatment should be started even with negative AFB and PCR, as delay in treatment can be devastating.

47. The answer is D. HIV-associated dementia is characterized by the classic triad of subcortical dementia: memory/psychomotor impairment, depression, and movement disorders. Seizure is not a typical component of this syndrome and should prompt an investigation of other processes. The dementia usually improved with initiation of antiretroviral therapy.

48. The answer is D. The patient has the dysarthria-clumsy hand syndrome, one of the 5 classic lacunar syndromes. Lacunar infarcts are caused by occlusion of a small penetrating branch of the larger cerebral vessels. Hypertension is the most important risk factor for lacunar infarctions. Dysarthria-clumsy hand syndrome is typically caused by occlusion of a penetrating branch to the pons, internal capsule' or corona radiata.

49. The answer is D. Dysarthria may be caused by a lesion in the primary motor cortex for the face, but it may also be from lesions anywhere in the corticobulbar tract. The other signs listed, however, represent deficits in higher cortical functions, the so-called "cortical localizing signs."

50. The answer is D. The patient most likely has postinfectious cerebellitis, or acute cerebellar ataxia. This syndrome is most common in children ages 2 to 7 years, and is rare in adults. It is characterized by acute cerebellar type ataxia that is maximal at onset. It is felt to be a postinfectious process, and frequently a preceding varicella infection is found on history. Treatment is supportive and most patients recover fully within days to weeks, but servere cases can take months to recover fully.

51. The answer is A. The patient most likely has trigeminal neuralgia. The symptoms most commonly involve the distribution of CN V-2 and V-3. Causes include MS (sometimes bilateral), mass lesions in the area of CN V such as meningioma or schwannoma in the cerebellopontine angle or brainstem, and, most commonly, microvascular compression of the nerve or nerve root. Giant cell arteritis typically affects older patients and causes pain in the area of the temporal artery.

52. The answer is **B**. The patient most likely has Lewy-body dementia. This is characterized by parkinsonian features such as rigidity and bradykinesia, as well as visual hallucinations and a fluctuating course of cognitive function. It is the second most common cause of dementia after Alzheimer's and likely represents some overlap between Alzheimer's and Parkinson's disease.

53. The answer is **E**. The patient's history is suggestive of dementia. While this is a chronic process and does not constitute an emergency, evaluating for reversible causes of dementia is a first step in the care of a patient with dementia. Thyroid dysfunction, B12 deficiency, neurosyphilis, normal pressure hydrocephalus, and CNS mass lesions are all potentially reversible causes of dementia. While rarely found to be the cause of dementia, they can be screened for with relatively low cost with the studies listed in choices A through D. A lumbar puncture is not indicated at this point in the work-up, but might be considered later if MRI suggested hydrocephalus as a cause or if neurosyphilis were suspected based on other data.

54. The answer is **E**. The patient has the alien hand syndrome in which one hand does not seem to belong to the patient. The most common lesion location for this syndrome is the corpus callosum. This is the extreme form of disconnection syndromes in which there is damage to the connections between different parts of the brain. Causes include mass lesions, multiple sclerosis, and infarctions.

55. The answer is **B**. The patient most likely has had a complicated migraine. It is hypothesized that migraines are accompanied by depolarization which may spread throughout the brain, sometimes causing focal neurologic signs such as weakness. Stroke and other structural lesions should always be ruled out before attributing focal signs to this phenomenon. The symptoms usually improve over hours to days. While thought to be benign in the sense that no infarction is found, there is an increased risk of infarction with use of triptans in these patients (thought to be because of vasoconstriction). This class of migraine medication should thus be avoided in patients with focal neurologic symptoms with their migraines.

56. The answer is **A**. The child likely has a medulloblastoma. It is a fast-growing primitive neuroectodermal tumor and is the most common primary brain tumor with onset in infancy. It is often located in the vermis or the fourth ventricle, and hydrocephalus is a common complication. Best results have been achieved when surgery, radiation, and chemotherapy are used in combination.

57. The answer is E. There are several possible reasons for the patient's weakness, including critical illness polyneuropathy, critical illness myopathy, steroid myopathy, and acute inflammatory demyelinating polyneuropathy. Stroke is unlikely given that all four limbs are involved. A cervical cord lesion could produce a quadriparesis, but without obvious trauma this is unlikely in this setting. Myasthenia can cause global weakness, but—like the disorders listed above—is best assessed acutely by EMG/nerve conduction studies, which can help distinguish myelopathic, myopathic, and neuropathic processes, as well as indicate whether neuropathic processes are axonal or demyelinating (important for prognosis).

58. The answer is C. Valproic acid is known to cause an idiopathic hyperammonemia in some patients. The mechanism seems to be disruption of the urea cycle. Patients may become encephalopathic from the elevated ammonia. Treatment includes carnitine administration, which shunts the urea cycle to increase metabolism of ammonia, and lactulose, which increases excretion of ammonia through the GI tract.

59. The answer is F. The patient has malignant hyperthermia, a life-threatening condition caused by neuromuscular blocking agents used in general anesthesia. It is often inherited in an autosomal dominant pattern and is thought to be a result of abnormal excitation-contraction coupling. The clinical effects include hyperthermia, rigidity, and metabolic acidosis because of muscle breakdown. Atropine should be avoided as it can cause hyperthermia.

60. The answer is A. The patient has restless legs syndrome. While the symptoms cause insomnia and can be associated with periodic limb movements of sleep, the primary problem is the irresistible urge to move the legs. Daily symptoms can be treated chronically with dopamine agonists such as pramipexole. Levodopa can be used intermittently, but leads to augmentation when used daily. Opiates and sedative-hypnotics are second-line agents.

61. The answer is A. The patient has Wilson's disease, characterized by Kayser-Fleischer rings, cirrhosis leading to splenomegaly, and neurological involvement with a parkinsonian picture. The disease is inherited in an autosomal recessive pattern, and involves abnormal binding of copper to its transport protein, leading to deposition in tissues, particularly the liver, brain, corneas, and kidneys. It can present with neurologic or hepatic symptoms, or both.

62. The answer is C. Lumbar puncture in multiple sclerosis typically reveals normal opening pressure, glucose, and protein/albumin. Leukocyte counts are usually less than 5 cells/mL. Slight elevations in these parameters are possible, but markedly abnormal findings should prompt investigation of other causes. Elevated IgG index and the presence of oligoclonal bands in CSF are suggestive of MS, but are not 100% specific. In conjunction with MRI findings, they help to make processes other than MS unlikely.

63. The answer is D. Lumbar puncture, performed properly by an experienced clinician, is a relatively benign procedure. By far the most common complication is a post-LP headache, which occurs in 20% to 30% of cases. The headache is typically mild and improved when lying flat (postural), and most cases resolve within hours to days. The incidence of post-LP headache is reduced by using smaller spinal needles with atraumatic tips. The other complications listed are exceedingly rare. Herniation does not occur unless there is a mass lesion causing increased intracranial pressure. Infection can be avoided by meticulous sterile technique. Bleeding disorders should be corrected prior to LP to avoid hematoma formation, but in emergency situations this is unnecessary.

64. The answer is I. Brain death criteria vary by institution and are dictated by state and local law. However, there are certain criteria common to brain death guidelines, and include known irreversible cause, ruling out metabolic complications, absence of hypothermia, ruling out intoxication, and an observation period that varies with the clinical situation. Clinical findings required to make the diagnosis include coma with no sign of cerebral-mediated response to noxious stimuli, absence of brainstem reflexes including caloric testing, and absence of spontaneous respiration as documented by apnea testing. In cases where any of these criteria are not met, ancillary or confirmatory tests may be performed to confirm the diagnosis. These include EEG to show absence of electrocerebral activity, cerebral angiography to document absence of intracerebral filling, or SPECT brain scan with absence of uptake. These latter tests are not necessary if the former criteria are met, but are useful in questionable cases.

65. The answer is D. The patient has subacute cerebellar degeneration, a paraneoplastic syndrome associated with breast, lung, and ovarian cancers in particular. While paraneoplastic disorders are a rare complication of cancer, when they occur they are often the presenting symptom. A positive paraneoplastic antibody test in the setting of a typical paraneoplastic syndrome is practically diagnostic, and a thorough search for underlying tumor should be sought. Biopsy of the cerebellum is unnecessary and often normal. Treatment includes treating the underlying tumor as well as immunosuppressive therapies, but the response is poor.

66. The answer is A. The patient has familial Parkinson's disease. Mutations in the α syncline gene have been linked to this disease, which leads to early onset parkinsonism. The other gene mutations listed are associated with other neurological diseases: NOTCH-3 is associated with CADASIL, SOD1 with ALS, Huntingtin with Huntington's disease, and DYT1 with dystonia.

67. The answer is A. Huntington's disease is inherited in an autosomal dominant pattern, so his son has a 50% chance of developing the disease. Because Huntington's disease is caused by a trinucleotide repeat, successive generations show anticipation, with earlier onset as the trinucleotide repeat is multiplied in each generation.

68. The answer is B. The patient likely has Wilson's disease, a disease of abnormal copper metabolism which results in copper deposits in the liver, brain, and other tissues. The characteristic Kayser-Fleischer rings are copper deposits in the Descemet membrane of the cornea. While the liver is typically the first organ affected, as many as 50% of patients present with neurological findings. The disease is autosomal dominant and is caused by mutation in a gene encoding a transmembrane copper transporting ATPase. Typical laboratory findings include decreased serum ceruloplasmin, increased 24-hour urine copper excretion, and increased hepatic copper content. Nonspecific findings include elevated liver enzymes. Serum copper concentrations are unreliable, as they may be low, normal, or elevated depending on the point in the disease process.

69. The answer is E. Spontaneous subarachnoid hemorrhage (SAH) is most commonly caused by rupture or an intracerebral aneurysm, sometimes by rupture of an arteriovenous malformation. Among the complications of SAH are continued bleeding, hydrocephalus, and cerebral vasospasm leading to infarction. Nimodipine, a relatively selective cerebral vasculature calcium channel blocker, has been shown to help prevent the delayed ischemic effects of SAH, presumably through a reduction in vasospasm of cerebral vessels.

70. The answer is D. The patient's symptoms of temporal headache and blurry vision are concerning for giant cell or temporal arteritis. This is a vasculitis of medium and large arteries which predominantly affects individuals over the age of 50 years. The most common presenting symptom is headache, with polymyalgia rheumatica, malaise, and jaw claudication among the other common symptoms. ESR is elevated in 97% of cases, with a mean value of 85. A normal ESR should thus push one to consider alternative diagnoses, while it does not exclude GCA. Temporal artery biopsy is the gold standard for diagnosis.

71. The answer is C. The constellation of headache, blurry vision, and seizure is not specific to any particular neurological process, but among the choices listed venous sinus thrombosis is the most likely to cause this syndrome. Giant cell arteritis and migraine are not typically associated with seizure. Stroke may rarely present with seizure, but would more likely lead focal neurological signs. Uncal herniation is excluded by the lack of decreased arousal. Because MS affects the white matter, it is not typically associated with seizure.

72. The answer is B. The patient has neurofibromatosis type 1 (NF 1) or von Recklinghausen's disease. This is the most common neurocutaneous syndrome. Cutaneous findings include multiple café-au-lait spots and axillary freckling, in addition to the neurofibromas that give the disease its name. Pigmented iris hamartomas called Lisch nodules are pathognomonic for NF 1. The most common CNS tumor associated with NF 1 is optic glioma; approximately 15% of patients with NF 1 have unilateral or bilateral optic glioma.

73. The answer is E. While many of the dementia syndromes eventually involve behavioral changes and language function, frontotemporal dementia in particular is characterized by derangements in behavior (personality changes, executive planning deficits) and in language (word-finding deficits, decreased speech output). This group of dementias is characterized by degeneration of the frontotemporal lobes out of proportion to other areas of the brain. It may be associated with motor neuron disease.

74. The answer is B. The patient has typical findings in dementia associated with Parkinson's disease, namely episodic memory impairments and executive dysfunction. Lewy bodies are the most consistent pathological finding, although senile plaques and neurofibrillary tangles are often seen as well, highlighting the overlap of Alzheimer's and Parkinson-type dementia.

75. The answer is A. The patient likely has early HIV-associated dementia. Early in the course, prominent features include subtle problems with memory, reading, math, or comprehension, as well as apathy and other depressive symptoms. As the process progresses, the classic syndrome includes global dementia, movement disorders, psychomotor slowing, and worsening depressive symptoms. Apathy may be treated with methylphenidate. At present, she does not have full-blown major depression, but antidepressants can be used if the syndrome is apparent. The most important treatment is proper anti-retroviral therapy, which this patient is already taking.

76. The answer is C. Most pediatric textbooks and many web sites for child development have tables of normal developmental milestones, often broken down by motor, sensory, and language/social skills. Many parents are concerned when their child does not do activities that other children the same age are able to do, or which their previous child was able to do at the same age. The important concept is that there is a range of ages for most developmental milestones, and children may achieve some goals during the normal age range or even ahead of normal, while having delays in other areas.

77. The answer is A. Hypertension is the single most important modifiable risk factor in primary stroke prevention. Smoking cessation, diabetes control, and reduction of elevated lipids are also important in primary prevention. Elevated homocysteine levels have been associated with increased risk for stroke, but therapies that are effective at lowering homocysteine levels have not been shown to change risk for stroke. Carotid artery stenosis is another significant modifiable risk factor for primary stroke prevention, and older patients and those with carotid bruits are sometimes screened for asymptomatic stenosis.

78. The answer is E. Hypercalcemia can cause mental status changes. Other electrolyte disturbances, which are known to cause altered mental status include hypernatremia, hyponatremia, and uremia. Work-up for any patient who presents with altered mental status should include screening chemistries, CBC, urinalysis, toxicology screen, and arterial blood gas.

79. The answer is B. Any patient suspected of having meningitis with rapidly worsening course should immediately receive broad coverage, CNS-penetrating antibiotics, including ceftriaxone, vancomycin, and ampicillin, as well as acyclovir to cover HSV. IV steroids have been shown to improve outcome, particularly in cases of pneumococcal meningitis, when given acutely with antibiotics. If there are neurological abnormalities, including depressed mental status, a head CT should be obtained to rule out hemorrhage or hydrocephalus. CSF will help narrow the diagnosis, but antibiotics should not be deferred to obtain an LP if a patient is rapidly worsening.

Once microbiology data are available, the treatment may be tailored to the particular infection.

80. The answer is A. The oculocephalic reflex is part of the coma examination, as no effort by the patient is required in order to perform the test. The patient's eyes are held open, and the head is passively rotated horizontally or vertically. A normal response in an unconscious patient is for conjugate (coordinated, synchronous) eye movement in the direction opposite the head movement, such that the eyes appear to fix on the examiner. This is a way to test that the eyes move in all four directions. If the eyes roll with the head, this "doll's eyes" response indicates a lesion somewhere in the pathway between labyrinth, vestibular nerve, medullary and pontine connections, or extraocular nerves or muscles. In a conscious patient, this reflex may be suppressed and so has less value. Note, this test should not be performed until a cervical spine injury is ruled out.

81. The answer is D. Temporal or giant cell arteritis is a vasculitis of medium to large-sized arteries. It is more common in patients older than 60 years of age, and four times more common in women than in men. Symptoms include headache, which may be unilateral, scalp tenderness over the temporal artery, jaw claudication, blurry vision, as well as systemic symptoms such as fever and joint pains (there is an association with polymyalgia rheumatica). Because of inflammation, ESR is almost uniformly elevated, often above 100. However, ESR is not 100% sensitive. C-reactive protein is another inflammatory marker that can support the diagnosis and be followed to access effectiveness of treatment. The gold standard diagnostic test is temporal artery biopsy. Note that in this case, the patient is already experiencing blurry vision. There is sufficient evidence to make the diagnosis, and treatment with steroids should not be postponed in order to obtain a biopsy, as the threat of vision loss dictates urgent treatment.

Index